NATURAL SOLUTIONS TO IBS

THE ULTIMATE GUIDE TO RELIEVING YOUR SYMPTOMS – FOR GOOD

MARILYN GLENVILLE
PhD

MACMILLAN

First published 2013 by Macmillan
an imprint of Pan Macmillan, a division of Macmillan Publishers Limited
Pan Macmillan, 20 New Wharf Road, London N1 9RR
Basingstoke and Oxford
Associated companies throughout the world
www.panmacmillan.com

ISBN 978-0-230-76922-9

1 3 5 7 9 8 6 4 2

A CIP catalogue record for this book is available from the British Library.

Text designed and set by seagulls.net
Printed and bound by CPI Group (UK) Ltd, Croydon, CR0 4YY

This book is intended as a reference volume only, not as a medical manual.
The information given here is designed to help you make informed decisions
about your health. It is not intended as a substitute for any treatment that you
may have been prescribed by your doctor. If you suspect you have a medical
problem, we urge you to seek competent medical help.

Visit **www.panmacmillan.com** to read more about all our books and to buy them.
You will also find features, author interviews and news of any author events, and you
can sign up for e-newsletters so that you're always first to hear about our new releases.

CONTENTS

ACKNOWLEDGEMENTS

I have wanted to write this book for quite a time, as IBS, which is often called a 'cinderella illness' because nobody pays any attention to it, affects the quality of life of so many people. Just because it is difficult to diagnose or used as a catch-all label for any digestive problems that can't conveniently be put in a medical 'box', it should not mean that it is ignored.

I would like to thank Liz Gough, my editor at Macmillan, who has been especially helpful in getting this book ready to be published. My thanks also go to Clare Hulton for introducing me to Macmillan and making this book possible.

I am grateful to Kate Adams who has helped to make sure that this book is easy to read and encouraged me to avoid getting too bogged down in the medical studies and technical terms.

I would especially like to thank my brilliant team of nutritionists, Alison Belcourt, Helen Heap, Sharon Pitt and Lisa Smith, who work in the London and Tunbridge Wells clinics and who take such good care of our patients. Thanks also go to the rest of the team in Tunbridge Wells, including Wendy, Brenda, Alex, Shirley, Kate, Sam, Mat, Lee and Dave, who work so diligently behind the scenes making the work I do possible. Particular thanks go to my two wonderful nutritionists in Ireland, Heather Leeson and Sally Milne, who are not

NATURAL SOLUTIONS TO IBS

only doing a superb job of looking after the women over there, but have also supplied many of the delicious recipes that are included in this book.

Very special thanks go to all my patients, who are really good in not 'putting up' with their IBS and have sought out a more holistic approach to the problem. Their feedback has been so helpful because, although the research and evidence in the medical literature is important, if it doesn't work in real life it is not helpful for people.

Last but not least, my love goes to my family: Kriss, my husband, and my three children Matt (and his wife Hannah, and their children Katie and Jack), Len and Chantell.

'It is more important to know what sort of person has a disease than to know what sort of disease a person has.'

Hippocrates

INTRODUCTION

Over the years I have seen patients with many different problems, from conditions like PCOS, endometriosis, fertility issues, problems arising from the menopause, and so much more. Most will come in with a confirmed diagnosis or I am able to suggest that they have certain tests or be referred to a specialist for scans or blood tests so they can get a diagnosis.

But Irritable Bowel Syndrome (IBS) is very different because there is no test, scan or procedure that can say you have it. IBS is a 'diagnosis of exclusion', meaning that other problems such as Crohn's or ulcerative colitis (or other digestive problems) are ruled out first until eventually you are left with the diagnosis of IBS. You are not alone if you get this diagnosis. It is estimated that up to one in five people are affected by IBS, with more women than men being diagnosed. There isn't enough research for a definitive answer as to why this is the case but it may be that women tend to seek out a diagnosis sooner than men or that female hormones have an exacerbating effect on the IBS symptoms (as I will explore in detail).

You should not feel alone if it has been a somewhat exhausting journey to get to your diagnosis. You may find that while you have a label for the symptoms you are experiencing, which in itself can be something of a relief, you may also have been told there is no definite cure for IBS. So where does that leave you and what do you do now? Live with the symptoms for the rest of your life? IBS is so often dismissed by the medical profession as a condition they can do little to help with. To me, this is unacceptable, because if you can find the cause of any problem then you can begin to treat it, and there is much we can do both to find the cause of IBS and then treat the symptoms.

Something is making your bowel 'irritable', and it is a question of trying to find out what that is while at the same time finding ways to help calm things down. IBS is described as a disorder in the way the bowel functions and so, in my view, it is important to try to work out just *why* your bowel is not functioning normally and use your diet and natural remedies to get your digestive system working well again.

You may not have reached the point of receiving a diagnosis of IBS, and have picked up this book to find out more about your digestive symptoms, for example you might suffer regularly from constipation and/or diarrhoea, flatulence or bloating. As you read through the book you will develop a good idea of how well your bowel is functioning and the tests that can help add a great deal more detail to the current picture. There is also plenty of practical advice to help establish good digestive health, because when your digestive system *is* working well you will reap a number of benefits, including better absorption of nutrients from your food, giving you more energy and improved general wellbeing. A stronger immune function, which is also one of the benefits of a healthy digestive system, will give your body the strength to fight off infections, and efficient detoxification ensures your body clears out and eliminates all the waste products and toxins that it should. You will feel lighter, healthier and symptom-free.

A DIFFERENT VIEW

The view from the medical side can often be negative, as seen in this quote about IBS from the *British Medical Journal*: 'The medical management of patients with IBS is often difficult. Doctors are still taught that IBS is a diagnosis of exclusion, and patients readily sense that they are being told that nothing is really wrong with them. Many people soon come to appreciate that the range of medical treatments available is limited in both scope and efficacy. The mood of negativity, once established, is difficult to dispel.'[1] I have met many patients who feel this is the case and often end up doing their own research into why they have these symptoms because they do not want to be fobbed off with a label – IBS – as if simply having the label makes everything alright. You may even have been told that it is psychosomatic because the doctors can't find anything physically wrong. Your mind is indeed powerful but if you are having very definite physical symptoms I would not suggest they are 'all in your mind'.

You may already have worked out that certain foods make the symptoms worse, and perhaps tried a number of different diets, but it's all rather confusing. You may have been given a medication to soothe your bowel but have had the realization that if the source of the irritability is not found you will be on this medication for life.

Most medical students will only receive a few hours of nutrition lectures in over six years of training, and yet it makes sense that a condition such as IBS will benefit the most from treatment through the diet. What you eat can have a profound effect on your health, and if you can give your body the right nutrients then you will give it the 'tools' to heal itself.

I wanted to write this book because IBS is the most common problem connected to the gastrointestinal tract and yet after a diagnosis, so many people are left wondering what they can do about it, and if they just have to put up with it. There are various ways to tackle IBS: it might be a case of finding out what is the right diet for you but, equally, there may be an underlying cause that has not been tracked down. The various tests available, which I outline in detail, will help identify the cause. For example, I remember a lovely lady coming into the clinic a few years back with a diagnosis of IBS and I suggested we do a stool test (see page 55 for more details on this test) to see how well her digestion was working, monitor her levels of beneficial bacteria and also to check for any parasites. The test showed that she had a parasite and on reflection she realized the IBS symptoms had developed after a trip to Egypt ten years ago when she had a bout of food poisoning. As soon as the parasites were dealt with, the 'IBS' disappeared.

I want to help you find the cause of your symptoms and give you natural solutions to alleviate them, because although people may suffer a similar combination of symptoms the causes may vary, and I think it is important to acknowledge that. I also want to help you stop IBS from affecting your quality of life so you don't have to plan each day around your condition. Perhaps you have stopped travelling to certain places because you are unsure whether there will be toilets close by – even going to the cinema or the theatre may be difficult unless you are sure you can get to the toilet quickly. This needn't be the case.

We will look at your whole body in relation to IBS, from how your digestive system is working, to the role that emotions and stress play with this condition. All the available medical and nutrition tests are explained, some of which can be extremely helpful. I will give you vital advice on how to support the digestive system, gently healing and strengthening it back to normal function with my Diet Plan, guidance on how to benefit from supplements, and I will also outline therapies for any anxiety or stress associated with your IBS. Using nutrition as a form of treatment works quite differently from conventional medicine. The first aim is to work on the symptoms by addressing the underlying cause of the problem. The next stage – and here's the big difference – is to work on *prevention*, because once you have addressed the root cause of the problem and know how to manage the condition, you often need only a simple maintenance programme to keep things on an even keel.

Step by step, we will nourish your digestion back to good health.

CASE STUDY: JANE'S STORY

I had always had what I would call 'normal' bowels and a healthy digestive system until two years ago when I changed job and worked as a PR consultant, putting in incredibly long stressful hours in the City. I would have diarrhoea at least once a day, which would be debilitating because of the pain, and it started to rule my life because I always had to be within reach of a toilet. This was incredibly difficult, especially when travelling or away from home and the office. To start with, it was difficult having to rush away from my desk at work during the day and it wasn't the easiest thing to talk about with my colleagues. However, I confided in a couple of people, making it slightly easier for me.

After a year of suffering I decided this wasn't normal and went to see my doctor who said it was just 'irritable bowel' and it was all in my mind and stress related. I went away feeling very upset and that I really hadn't been listened to. He prescribed me a drug to stop the diarrhoea but I knew this was only masking the underlying problem. I took the course of medication for a month but had such bad cramps and bloating that I decided to stop taking it. I went back to my doctor and he referred me to a gastroenterologist (reluctantly!). I had an endoscopy and colonoscopy which both came back 'normal', yet I knew it was not normal to have such chronic symptoms.

I was talking to a colleague at work who mentioned that she had been to see a nutritionist for her digestive problems. She had been experiencing constipation and bloating and, within a month, she was a different person. She gave me the number of the Dr Marilyn Glenville Clinic and I phoned straight away. Before booking an appointment, a nutritionist at the clinic spoke with me to make sure my problem was something that could be helped by nutrition. She explained that my symptoms came under the 'umbrella' of irritable bowel syndrome and it was certainly influenced by diet but stress could exacerbate it. She briefly mentioned the common trigger foods that I may have to cut out and although it sounded hard I was desperate to feel well again so I booked the appointment.

My first consultation lasted one hour and the nutritionist took a very detailed history and went through my 'typical' diet – something that the doctor never did because he said that it was nothing to do with food. She explained that IBS differs from other bowel disorders like Crohn's and colitis in that there is no underlying detectable pathology (i.e. nothing shows up with routine medical investigation) that is causing the digestive symptom or discomfort. However, as the name suggests, there must be something that is causing an irritation to the bowel. Commonly acknowledged foods that irritate the intestinal wall include dairy products, coffee, alcohol, wheat and citrus fruits. Well, this was my diet! I would drink a couple of cappuccinos to get me through my stressful working day and lived on sandwiches and biscuits washed down with orange juice!

The nutritionist talked about stress and how it impacts on digestion. When the body is under stress the energy available to the digestive tract is compromised so the release of digestive enzymes – naturally produced by our body to help digest carbohydrates, fats and proteins – is impaired and food is not digested properly, resulting in diarrhoea and bloating. It all made so much sense because stress definitely made my symptoms worse – almost like an 'exam tummy' churning around. I thought this was something I just had to live with because of the nature of my job. From my experience, stress and IBS became a vicious cycle because my stress would trigger my symptoms and my painful bloating and diarrhoea made me more stressed, and so on.

I cut out all bread, pasta, biscuits and cereals and, of course, my milky cappuccinos and cheese. However, much to my amazement, I found some great alternatives, readily available from the supermarket, that made my life easier. Even eating out at restaurants I became aware of so many wheat- and dairy-free options. I suppose until you have to avoid certain foods, you don't look to see what else is out there.

The nutritionist also suggested basic vitamins and minerals to boost my immune system plus specific gut support in the form of a probiotic, to boost all the 'friendly' bacteria living throughout my digestive system, and digestive enzymes that I had to take specifically every time I ate to help digest the food and reduce my bloating.

Within four days my diarrhoea had stopped and consequently I no longer had a painful bloated stomach. For the first time in years I wasn't constantly thinking about having to find a toilet and my commute to and from work was stress-free. My clothes felt comfortable at the end of the day and I didn't look six months pregnant as I often did before I went to the clinic. I couldn't believe how such common foods could cause such debilitating symptoms. For the first time I was actually enjoying my food and taking a real interest in what I was putting into my body rather than just stuffing a sandwich down every lunchtime and relying on that coffee fix to get me through the day.

I had my follow-up consultation four weeks later and the nutritionist recommended I continue with the same diet for another eight weeks, after which I could try reintroducing one food at a time. She explained that I may be able to eat these foods in moderation in the future, but for the moment it was important just to keep the digestive system calm and not stress it with foods that it was trying to 'fight'. This made so much sense, plus I was motivated because I felt so well, so naturally wanted to continue.

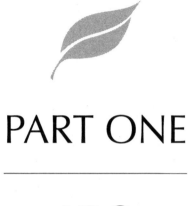

PART ONE

IBS

CHAPTER 1

WHAT IS IBS?

IBS is the most common problem associated with the digestive system. It is classed as a syndrome because it is a collection of different symptoms and you can have most or just a few of these symptoms in varying extremes of discomfort.

IBS affects up to 20 per cent of the population, with women most commonly affected. It is defined as 'a chronic, relapsing, gastrointestinal problem, characterized by abdominal pain, bloating and changes in bowel habit' and ranks as high as the common cold in terms of people needing days off work to cope with it.[1]

SYMPTOMS

Not everyone gets the same symptoms but the most common ones include:

- Abdominal discomfort/pain/cramps or spasms
- Diarrhoea
- Constipation
- Alternating constipation or diarrhoea

- Bloating
- Gas/flatulence and rumbling noises in the intestines
- Heartburn or indigestion
- Nausea
- Relief on passing stools
- Mucous/jelly-like substance in stools
- Frequent toilet visits – both for passing urine as well as bowel motions
- Tiredness and lethargy
- Headaches
- Sleep problems
- Back pain
- Period pains
- PMS
- Pain during intercourse for women

In addition to the physical symptoms above, IBS can also affect you mentally with emotional symptoms that include:

- Mood swings
- Hopelessness
- Depression
- Anxiety

IBS highlights just how strong the mind–body connection is. Scientists even call the gut the 'second brain' because it is filled with neurotransmitters we usually associate with being in the brain. Our brain and gut are therefore intimately connected and that's why they can affect each other so much. Anxiety gives most people butterflies in the stomach, and for those with IBS anxiety can trigger the onset of symptoms such as constipation, cramps or diarrhoea. And it works both ways, because the physical symptoms of IBS can trigger strong emotions, setting up a pattern that is often difficult to break free from. This is why I have found that the holistic approach of my treatment plan for IBS can work so well for people, as once you begin to alleviate the symptoms through your diet and identify triggers, you can then begin to feel better both physically and emotionally. IBS can be very draining for people, and they may feel either mentally exhausted or constantly on high alert. Once you can begin to feel more at ease in your body you set up a more positive pattern both with food and your outlook on life in general (see Chapter 7 for more on the emotional side of IBS).

Researchers have tried to classify people suffering from IBS into three groups:

- Those where the diarrhoea is more predominant (IBS-D), which accounts for about one third of IBS sufferers
- Those where constipation is more predominant (IBS-C), which again affects about one third
- Those where the bowel motions can be mixed, or alternate between diarrhoea and constipation (sometimes called IBS-A or IBS-M)

The difficulty is that the research doesn't always split up the types when discussing beneficial treatments so it can be hard to establish which treatments are going to be most effective for each type. Over time many sufferers can also switch between types, and people with constipation or diarrhoea can develop an alternating pattern of bowel motions.[2]

You will find that many of the dietary suggestions and remedies recommended in this book will apply no matter what type of IBS you have. But I have also included a separate chapter at the end (see Chapter 8) that focuses on particular symptoms, so you can get more individual help with specific problems.

WHAT IS NOT IBS?

As mentioned, IBS is a diagnosis of exclusion so if you've received your diagnosis you should already have had tests to rule out any major problems, and I will cover these in Chapter 2.

When these tests show that your digestive system is normal then you are given the diagnosis of IBS. This means that there is no change in the actual structure of your gastrointestinal tract, ruling out the group of Inflammatory Bowel Diseases (IBD) that includes Crohn's and ulcerative colitis. IBD can often be confused with IBS, but with IBD there is evident inflammation in the gut and it is thought to be an autoimmune problem. With IBS the bowel is normal in structure; the problem lies with how it functions. You can also rest assured that having IBS does not increase your risk of bowel cancer. There is no immediately obvious cause for the symptoms, hence the difficulty doctors often have in treating the condition, but there is much you can do to help identify the root cause, triggers and alleviate irritation.

WHAT CAUSES IBS?

We don't yet know the exact causes but there have been a number of theories suggested and it can be different for each person so I always work individually with patients to find their root cause. As you read through the book I hope you will also be able to detect the initial trigger for your IBS as it can be so helpful in finding the best treatments for your own symptoms.

It is thought a stressful event such as divorce, accident or bereavement can trigger the onset of IBS. If you recognize that this might be the case for you then it is as important to pay close attention to the chapter on emotions (Chapter 7) as it is to focus on your diet (Chapter 5).

Another theory is that IBS is triggered by a gastrointestinal infection or food poisoning, as research shows that you are twice as likely to develop IBS after having an attack of gastroenteritis.[3] This is why the healing attributes of pro- and prebiotics can be so helpful for IBS (see pages 132–4).

In some people the nerves and muscles in the bowel may be extra sensitive and can react when eating so that when the bowel stretches there is pain and spasms. In this case we look to calm the gut with non-irritating foods that are comforting and healing

Research shows that taking a course of antibiotics can increase the risk of developing IBS by more than three times.[4] We also now know that children prescribed at least one course of antibiotics by the time they are four are twice as likely to develop IBS.[5]

Sensitivity or allergies to certain foods have also been suggested as a trigger (see pages 44–50). When this is the case I often find an exclusion diet (see page 65) is the best way to find out which foods are triggering your IBS symptoms. Once you've identified them, sometimes it is a case of steering clear of these foods forever, but I often find that over time patients can begin to introduce them back in gradually as their gut heals and strengthens.

For some patients we discover their trigger is a yeast overgrowth, known as Candida albicans (see page 51), that then creates symptoms associated with IBS.

And for women, some believe that there may be an interaction between the bowels and the female hormones. This theory is based on the fact that many women experience worse IBS symptoms during menstruation (see below).

DIFFERENCES BETWEEN MEN AND WOMEN WITH IBS

Three times more women than men are diagnosed with IBS and they are five times more likely to seek help for the symptoms.[6] We don't know for sure whether more women actually suffer from IBS, or if they are just more likely to go to their doctors for help. Women may be more sensitive to pain or may be less willing to put up with the pain than men, or it is thought perhaps that women are more prone to stress and anxiety, which may increase IBS symptoms (see Chapter 7). For women, it tends to be the symptom of abdominal pain that impacts quality of life so significantly, followed by gas and bloating.[7]

Hormones may play a part as women will often experience worsening IBS symptoms during the pre-menstrual time of the month and particularly during menstruation. Women without IBS commonly have looser stools during their period but women with IBS will also often have more frequent bowel motions, increased pain and bloating and generally feel less well.[8] Going through hormonal changes may affect how women perceive pain as there seem to be more women diagnosed with IBS during their teens and early twenties and then their fifties, during the perimenopause.[9] And the fact that taking HRT (Hormone Replacement Therapy) for menopausal symptoms can increase the risk of having IBS does seem to confirm that the influence of female hormones may be a factor.[10] Current and past users of HRT were found to be at increased risk of IBS compared to women of the same age who had never used HRT. The risk was there no matter how long the women had taken HRT or in what form (pills or patches).

We know men tend to suffer more with looser stools than women, whereas female symptoms tend to veer more towards constipation with harder, lumpier stools. This could be explained by the fact that the female hormones, oestrogen and progesterone, slow down the progress of food through the digestive tract, making constipation more common for women. This also explains why many women have told me that they get diarrhoea as their period comes because that is when oestrogen and progesterone drop, ready to start the next menstrual cycle.

This drop in the hormones produced by the ovaries just before the period also explains why there can be a general increase in gastrointestinal symptoms including abdominal pain, discomfort and bloating around this time, and the same increase in symptoms can happen in the lead up to the menopause (the perimenopause) when the ovarian hormones are also decreasing.[11] Period pains (dysmenorrhea) and IBS are often connected, with women IBS sufferers more likely to experience period pains. PMS symptoms are also worse in women who also have IBS,[12] and it seems that IBS symptoms can increase after the menopause.[13] Added to this is that women with endometriosis can have many of the gastrointestinal symptoms that are usually associated with IBS including diarrhoea and bloating.

And just as hormones can affect digestion, so the digestive system can also have a direct impact on the female hormones. The liver deals with oestrogen and converts it into a less harmful form so it can be eliminated safely from the body. After being changed into an inactive form by the liver, oestrogen then passes into the bowel. As long as the levels of bacteria in the bowel are good then oestrogen is excreted safely out through the faeces. But if there is dysbiosis (an imbalance of good and bad bacteria) in the gut then the oestrogen can end up being converted back into the active form and recirculated in the blood. So a woman can end up with a dominance of oestrogen because her body is not detoxifying it efficiently. Some women's health problems, such as fibroids, endometriosis and certain breast cancers, are oestrogen sensitive so digestive health is crucial for keeping hormones in balance.

Recent research also shows that there can be an increased risk of miscarriage and ectopic pregnancy in women who suffer from IBS so it is vital that you tackle your IBS by following the recommendations in this book, especially if you are a woman and planning to get pregnant.[14]

CASE STUDY: CAROLE

Carole, thirty-seven, came to one of my clinics with symptoms of bloating, wind, irregular bowel movements, being prone to stomach upsets, having difficulty in digesting fatty foods, constipation and extreme pain when passing a bowel motion. She had been experiencing these symptoms since she was seventeen. Carole had previously been diagnosed with endometriosis and had had surgery for this but she knew that her bowel symptoms were much worse when she was having a period.

My nutritionist recommended Carole do a stool test and this showed that she had an imbalance between the good and negative bacteria in the gut, two different types of yeast, a parasite and very low levels of Secretory IgA (an antibody that provides the first line of defence in the gut against bacteria, yeasts and problem foods).

Carole was advised to eliminate gluten, dairy foods and soya from her diet. She was put on a programme of supplements, which included a good multivitamin and mineral, Omega 3 fish oils, probiotics and other nutrients to eliminate the yeast and parasite.

By her third appointment Carole was much improved, she was emptying her bowels every day without pain and the bloating and wind had reduced considerably. By the fourth appointment Carole felt really good and felt that the IBS was under control. She was happy to keep to a no gluten, no soya and no dairy diet as it kept her symptoms under control.

Carole repeated the stool test in three months' time to check the change in bacteria and parasites and then her programme of supplements was altered accordingly. She was also advised to continue taking the multivitamin and mineral (which contains calcium to offset the loss from the no-dairy diet) and also the Omega 3 fish oils. Over time, Carole may be able to introduce some gluten containing foods, dairy or soya in small quantities.

YOUR DIGESTIVE SYSTEM

Anyone who suffers from IBS will know exactly what I mean when I say that your digestive system 'isn't functioning normally'. I think it's helpful, therefore, to examine the digestive process from start to finish and look at how everything should be working when all is well.

Think of your digestive system as a long tube from your mouth to your anus. Your food goes on a 29-foot (9-metre) journey from start to finish; it goes in one end, is processed and the goodness extracted and then the waste is pushed out the other end. It also functions as an essential barrier separating your gut from the rest of your body. And although your digestive system is a tube-like cylinder from one end to the other, if you were to unfold it, the surface area would be the size of two tennis courts because of the folds within the surface. The cells within your digestive system renew themselves quite rapidly, about every four days.

YOUR MOUTH

As you chew, your mouth is performing the first part of the digestion process. Most people tend to think that the stomach is the first part of digestion and might swallow their food quite quickly without chewing it very much at all. However, the act of chewing, or mastication as it is known medically, does two really important things. Firstly, the mechanical action of chewing breaks your food down into smaller particles, which makes it easier to be processed, but also these smaller pieces of food come into contact with the enzymes contained in your saliva. The carbohydrates you eat start their digestion in your mouth when they are broken down by the salivary enzyme alpha-amylase, and the fats also start being digested by the enzyme lipase, which is secreted by glands under your tongue.

Secondly, chewing is the signal to the rest of your digestive system that food is on its way. Once you swallow your food, it passes into your oesophagus (gullet) in order to make the journey into your stomach.

YOUR STOMACH

Your stomach is a bag of acid (strong enough to dissolve a razor blade!) and performs a number of vital digestive functions. It can store food, so that if you have a large meal your stomach can hold it and deal with the breakdown of that food over time. It also breaks food down; a combination of the strong hydrochloric acid, protein-digesting enzymes and muscular churning of the stomach turns the food into a liquid mixture called chyme. The stomach then slowly releases the chyme into the small intestines. It takes about four hours for the whole contents of your stomach to be emptied into your small intestines.

THE SMALL INTESTINES

This is the part of your bowel that does the most work in terms of digestion. Your pancreas secretes digestive enzymes which work on breaking down carbohydrates, fats and proteins. When the food has been digested, the nutrients are passed into the blood vessels in the intestinal walls and then they can be carried around your body by your blood supply to the various organs. About half of the contents of the your small intestines will have emptied into your large intestines over three hours.

THE LARGE INTESTINES

This is the other part of your bowel, also known as your colon, and its role is to absorb water from the indigestible waste in order to produce

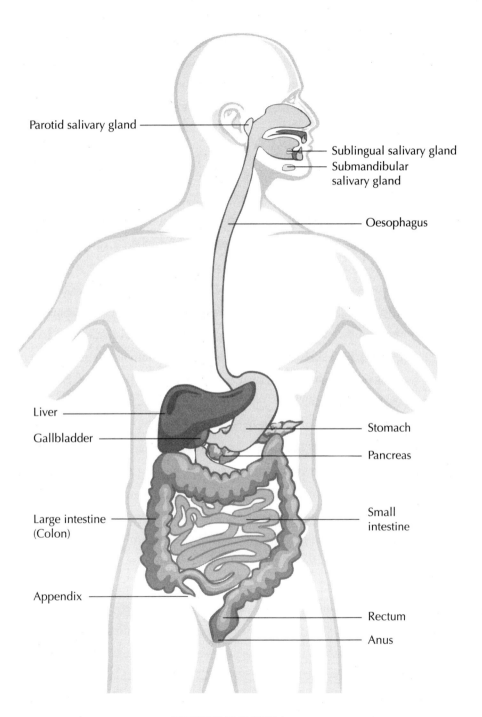

DIGESTIVE SYSTEM

faeces, which are excreted out of your body by muscle contractions called peristalsis. You might think it's only a day between eating and excreting the waste from that food, but the journey through this part of your digestive system takes about thirty to forty hours.

BENEFICIAL BACTERIA

Both your small and large intestines are host to millions of beneficial bacteria. The human body is host to around 100,000,000,000,000 bacteria – that's around 1kg (2lb) in weight. Having good levels of beneficial bacteria is important for all these reasons:

- Improved nutrition – the 'good' bacteria help to manufacture nutrients like the B vitamins, including folic acid, and also vitamin K, which helps with normal blood clotting. The bacteria can also help with the efficient digestion of food, especially protein, which can reduce the possibility of an allergy.
- Immune benefits – the beneficial bacteria can help to ward off and even kill 'negative' bacteria. They can help to control yeasts such as candida (see page 51).
- Improved detoxification – by aiding digestion the beneficial bacteria stop food sitting in the gut and producing toxins when it putrefies. They also help the body eliminate hormones such as oestrogen through the digestive system.

Lactobacillus acidophilus is the main species of beneficial bacteria that colonizes the small intestines while the bifidobacterium are the main beneficial inhabitants of the large intestines.

Unfortunately, the levels of these beneficial bacteria can be easily altered by certain factors. Taking certain drugs such as antibiotics, steroids, the Pill or HRT will reduce the levels of 'good' bacteria and

MEDICATIONS AND IBS

It is worth making sure that any medication you may be taking is not causing or intensifying your IBS symptoms. Many medications can affect the digestive system, and as your digestive system is already sensitive and irritable the effects may be much stronger.

Some of the well-known medications that cause IBS symptoms, such as constipation or diarrhoea, include painkillers (especially those containing codeine), antibiotics, iron (especially ferrous sulphate), drugs used to treat anxiety (like amitriptyline), some drugs used to treat high cholesterol (like cholestyramine), drugs for high blood pressure (calcium-channel blockers), diuretics, non-steroidal anti-inflammatory drugs used for problems such as arthritis, anti-histamines and also some antidepressants.

More than 700 drugs have been implicated in causing diarrhoea and it may not be the drug itself but an ingredient like lactose or sorbitol used in the tablet that may be the culprit.[15] Or there could be an artificial sweetener or colour added to the drug which is triggering digestive problems for you.

You may now realize that your 'IBS' started when you went on a certain medication or when you changed to a different drug. Obviously you need to speak to your doctor if you suspect that a medication you are taking can be causing or worsening your IBS symptoms and if you need to take that medication then maybe there is a different type you could have instead. Also have a look at the drug leaflet to check the other ingredients in case it is simply an added ingredient that is the trigger – again, your doctor may be able to prescribe a different one.

a diet high in fat, sugar, alcohol and too little fibre will also do the same. Stress can alter this delicate balance, as can travelling abroad, food poisoning (being infected by salmonella for example) and the levels will, in addition, naturally decline as you get older. In Chapter 6, How to Use Supplements and Herbs, I have included probiotics and prebiotics, plus in the Diet Plan there are plenty of food sources of these wonderful digestive helpers.

BOWEL MOTIONS

You should be passing a bowel motion at least once a day. Some patients in the clinic think that 'regular' means every three days; it does not. It is also good to get into the habit of having a bowel motion first thing in the morning. This will cause your body to automatically send messages to your colon for a stool to be pushed towards the back passage, ready to be defecated each morning (see page 186). Following the practical advice and the plan in this book will help you educate your body in this way as it is so helpful for developing digestive health.

It is also important to be aware of what your stools look like. To help you judge what is 'normal', there is a system of classifying bowel motions called the Bristol Stool Form Scale.[16] The scale is divided into seven categories:

1. Separate hard lumps, like nuts (hard to pass)
2. Sausage shaped, but lumpy
3. Like a sausage or snake, but with cracks on the surface
4. Like a sausage or snake, smooth and soft
5. Soft blobs with clear-cut edges (easy to pass)
6. Fluffy pieces with ragged edges, a mushy stool
7. Water, no solid pieces, liquid

We are aiming for types 3 and 4, the ideal bowel motions. Types 1 and 2 are classed as constipation and from 5 to 7 you are moving towards diarrhoea.

So the digestive system is both amazing and complex; when it is working well it's our source of energy and even our vitality. But with so much happening during the process, perhaps it's no wonder that so many people find their own digestion is out of balance, especially with modern diets and lifestyles.

It is very useful to get a good picture of the whole digestive system so we can begin to detect where the problem might lie. It might not be the underlying cause but even how you are eating, for example, can certainly exacerbate your symptoms, literally from the moment (and even before) food enters your mouth. Think about how you eat. Be honest; perhaps you are in the habit of eating very fast, swallowing food before you have fully chewed it? Or perhaps you have a habit of eating in front of the TV, so your stomach is squashed, which doesn't help digestion? Or you may have a yeast problem as yet undetected, or not enough beneficial bacteria, so your food is producing too many toxins in your gut. Or perhaps there are specific foods that irritate a particular part of the process and so produce painful symptoms such as spasms and flatulence. Or your mind could be literally stressing your stomach out, further disrupting normal service.

Think about what might have been the initial trigger for your IBS when it first came about. Can you link it back to a stressful or very traumatic event in your life? Or might there be a physical cause, such as a bad case of food poisoning? Perhaps you literally felt weakened by this and your digestion never quite recovered. Think carefully about the possible root cause of your problem.

In the next chapter we look in more detail at how IBS might be diagnosed, because this diagnosis will give us very helpful signs for how to treat and alleviate the symptoms.

CHAPTER 2

DIAGNOSING IBS

How do you get a diagnosis of IBS when there is no blood test or scan that can confirm it? This has been a dilemma in the medical world for many years and it is only in the last decade or so that the spotlight has been put on IBS and how to diagnose it.

There isn't yet a definitive diagnosis, but in the past ten to fifteen years a number of criteria have been proposed so that doctors can have a checklist of symptoms that can help to guide the diagnosis. You might not feel it's very comprehensive but it's useful to know just what kind of criteria your doctor is likely to be looking for.

THE ROME III CRITERIA FOR IBS

In the US there is the Rome III Criteria (2006) by the Rome Foundation, a not-for-profit organization that aims to improve the diagnosis and treatment of functional gastrointestinal disorders of which IBS is one (see www.romecriteria.org). There have been number I and II Criteria in the past, which goes to show how the diagnosis changes over time. The Rome III Criteria is: recurrent abdominal pain or discomfort at least three days during the month in the last three months associated with two or all of the following and the onset of symptoms at least six months prior to diagnosis:

1. Improvement with defecation
2. Onset associated with a change in frequency of stool
3. Onset associated with a change in form (appearance) of stool

NICE CRITERIA FOR IBS

In the UK, NICE (National Institute for Clinical Excellence, www. nice.org.uk) has also published criteria (2008) for the diagnosis of IBS. And they have used the first three letters of the alphabet to make an easy-to-see checklist:

A   Abdominal pain or discomfort
B   Bloating
C   Change in bowel habit

You must have had any one or more of the above symptoms for at least six months. This is then followed up with more detailed criteria:

Consider a positive diagnosis of IBS only if the person complains of abdominal pain or discomfort that is either relieved by defecation or associated with altered bowel frequency or altered stool form. This pain or discomfort must also be accompanied by at least two of the following four symptoms (other features such as lethargy, nausea, backache and bladder symptoms are common in people with IBS and may be used to support the diagnosis).

1. *Altered stool passage (straining, urgency, incomplete evacuation)*
2. *Abdominal bloating (less common in men than women), distension, tension or hardness*
3. *Symptoms made worse by eating*
4. *Passage of mucus*

The guidelines recommend that if you meet the above criteria that you are then given the following blood tests to ensure there is not another medical problem causing your symptoms. I have listed these below because if you have been given the diagnosis of IBS from just your symptoms it is important that you have these tests in order to rule out any other problems. (If you have difficulties getting these blood tests done then do contact my clinic – see Useful Resources, page 207.)

1. Full blood count – this will look at the kinds and number of different cells in your blood including red and white blood cells and platelets.
2. Erythrocyte sedimentation rate (ESR) or plasma viscosity – both of these can indicate inflammation.
3. C reactive protein – a measure of inflammation that can indicate problems such as inflammatory bowel disease or rheumatoid arthritis.
4. Antibody testing for coeliac disease – to rule out problems with gluten, which is the protein in a number of grains (see page 57 for more on coeliac disease).

RED FLAG INDICATORS

Because the diagnosis of IBS is one of exclusion, it is important that any other possible problem that might give you the same symptoms is ruled out. There are a number of symptoms which are given a 'red flag', meaning that if you have any of these you should be referred on to a specialist for further investigations. I have listed these below and it is important that you stress these to your doctor if you are experiencing them.

The red flag symptoms include:

1. Unintentional and unexplained weight loss
2. Rectal bleeding
3. A recent change in bowel habit to looser and/or more frequent stools that has persisted for more than six weeks in a patient aged over sixty years
4. A family history of bowel or ovarian cancer

The blood tests and the red flag indicators aim to rule out any other medical problems such as:

*   Inflammatory Bowel Disease (including Crohn's and ulcerative colitis)
*   Ovarian cancer
*   Endometriosis
*   Diverticulitis
*   Bowel cancer

The NICE guidelines state that the following tests are not needed to confirm a diagnosis of IBS if you meet all the other criteria. These tests below are only used to rule out any other diagnosis, leaving IBS as the only diagnosis left.

1. Ultrasonography – scanning using ultrasound
2. Sigmoidoscopy – camera inserted into the anus to examine the last third of your large intestines
3. Colonoscopy – camera inserted into the anus to look at the whole length of your large intestines
4. Barium enema – X-ray to check your bowels
5. Thyroid function blood test
6. Stool test for parasites

I wanted to discuss the tests in detail so you know you have had all the correct tests and to help you feel confident that you now have an accurate diagnosis. If you think that there are tests missing that you should have had then do go back to your doctor to discuss this, or you are welcome to contact my clinic as following a consultation we can give you a referral to see a private gastroenterologist if need be (see Useful Resources, page 207).

Once you have a diagnosis your doctor can explore the medical options with you, which I will go through in detail in the next chapter so that you can be fully aware of the treatments now available. In my thirty years of experience I know how vital diet and nutrition are, both in alleviating IBS symptoms and often in discovering the cause of the condition, for example a food intolerance or parasite from a bout of food poisoning. I would always encourage anyone to take a nutritional approach to IBS in the first instance, but as this can take a bit of time for the effects to really be felt you might want to think about the medical options too. Always talk things through with your doctor and go with what feels right for you.

CHAPTER 3

YOUR MEDICAL OPTIONS

So you've been told you have IBS, and now you want to know what medical options are available to you. As IBS is a problem to do with how your bowel is functioning rather than a 'structural' problem I would always encourage you to follow the nutritional recommendations in Chapter 5. Having said that, I do understand that for some of you the symptoms may have been affecting the quality of your life for so long that you are desperate to see and feel results. Dietary changes do usually take longer to have an impact and there is no reason not to combine the medical choices with the nutritional recommendations. As you start to feel confident that your symptoms are improving, you can talk to your doctor to see about either reducing the dose of the medication or stopping it completely.

I will outline the different medications you might be offered, how successful they are according to the research and what side effects you might experience.

You may be offered drugs to alter transit time of food through the digestion system. So, to slow things down if you have diarrhoea or to speed things up a little if you have constipation. Other drugs can be used to reduce pain and bloating or to relax the muscles in your gut and therefore relieve spasms. You may be offered a combination of drugs to tackle a number of the symptoms at the same time and how successful the medication might be varies enormously from person to person so don't be disheartened if you don't see immediate results.

NICE (National Institute for Clinical Excellence) suggests that the first medications that you should be offered, either on their own or in combination, would be antispasmodics (along with dietary and lifestyle advice which I will cover in Chapters 5 and 6), laxatives if you are constipated, loperamide (an antimotility agent) if you have diarrhoea and to adjust the dosages of the laxative or antimotility until you have a stool which is soft and well-formed and would be a number 4 on the Bristol Stool Form Scale (see page 24).

MEDICATIONS FOR IBS: THE LATEST RESEARCH

Unfortunately, so far, the failure rate for medical treatments of IBS seems to be high.[1] What is also interesting is that the placebo effect in clinical trials of IBS is very high at almost 50 per cent, so when people suffering from IBS are given a dummy pill they report feeling better.[2] This makes it difficult to determine just how effective the drug is compared to the placebo in a clinical trial. But it also means that there could be a psychological element to some of the symptoms of IBS and I will cover this in Chapter 7, including how to address any emotional triggers.

I want to stress that this does not mean you are 'making it all up' or that it is 'all in your mind'. There are strong links between the brain and the gut, so much so the gut is often called your 'second brain'. It has its own complex nervous system and also, just like your brain, produces serotonin, the 'feel good' neurotransmitter.

It is likely that for people taking part in a clinical trial with IBS, this could be the first time that somebody has taken their symptoms seriously. It is interesting that research shows that people are often left feeling unhappy with their doctors and other healthcare providers (HCPs) when it comes to their treatment and management of IBS. Over 50 per cent of people thought their relationship with their doctor was negative and comments included 'I don't trust my HCP' and 'my HCP thinks I'm crazy', although some said 'my HCP has been helpful and reassuring'. The conclusion of the research was largely negative, with major concerns that people were not being listened to properly and not feeling any empathy from their HCP.[3]

So when enrolling in a clinical trial, regardless of whether the person is on the active drug treatment or on the placebo, they will be listened to regarding their symptoms and time will have been spent with them. The sense of relief this must create could be 'transmitted' to the bowel and so could account for the high placebo response.

The placebo effect also increases depending on the frequency of the interaction between the doctor and the patient. It has been suggested that rather than seeing the placebo effect as being something negative, it could instead be used to good effect and actually help people get more relief from their IBS symptoms.[4]

ANTI-SPASMODIC DRUGS

These work by relaxing the muscles in your bowel and stopping the spasms which can cause pain. They have been shown to be effective for IBS and are often used to treat flare-ups of pain, or are taken regularly before food if the pain starts soon after eating.[5] Different brands of antispasmodics can include mebeverine and hyoscine.

Side effects can include allergic reactions including swelling of the lips, tongue or face or red rash with itching. For hyoscine there can be an increase in heart rate (tachycardia) and dry mouth and there can also be changes in vision which may affect your ability to drive, and loss of vision or seeing haloes, which means there can be increased pressure inside the eyeball and you need to see your doctor immediately.

LAXATIVES

You may be offered laxatives if constipation is a major problem for you. I will cover the more 'natural' laxatives in Chapter 6, but will discuss the most commonly medically recommended laxatives here.

Laxatives can work in a number of ways and some are really unsuitable for IBS. The ones to avoid with IBS are the stimulant laxatives.

STIMULANT LAXATIVES

These kinds of laxatives work by irritating the lining of the bowel, which causes muscle contractions to move the stool along. These are meant to be used only in the short term because you can end up becoming dependent on them, which means the bowel becomes lazy and so you need higher and higher doses to get the same effect. Examples of this kind of laxative include senna and bisacodyl. Ironically, side effects can include stomach cramping, diarrhoea and vomiting.

BULK-FORMING LAXATIVES

These are supplements of plant fibre and can include bran, ispaghula (also known as psyllium) husks and methylcellulose. They increase stool frequency by adding water and bulk to the stool.

Research shows that there is no evidence that these bulking agents are helpful for IBS[6] and, ironically, side effects (especially with bran) can include more abdominal pain, bloating and flatulence.[7] The best one of these to try would be the ispaghula (psyllium husks) – see how you get on with it. But I would definitely suggest you avoid bran.

OSMOTIC LAXATIVES

These kinds of laxative work by holding water in your colon which softens the stools and makes them easier to pass out. Different versions include lactulose and macrogols.

Side effects can include diarrhoea, bloating and dehydration.

ANTI-DIARRHOEAL DRUGS

If your major problem is diarrhoea rather than constipation, then you may be offered medication to help stop this. The usual treatment is to prescribe loperamide, which helps to slow down the movement of the stool through your gut and also allows more time for the stool to harden and form. Loperamide can also help with that feeling of urgency, and may stop leakage, which can be more common at night. It does work for people with diarrhoea from IBS, but does not help with any associated pain.

You would need to experiment with the dose of this medication because it can end up working too well, giving you constipation, and you don't want to then end up taking laxatives to solve that problem, obviously.

Side effects can include abdominal cramps, bloating, drowsiness, dizziness and skin rashes. Cramps and bloating are symptoms of IBS, so you don't want to end up making your symptoms worse. I would suggest you use these medications with caution and speak to your doctor if you experience any of these symptoms.

The important point to remember about these medications is that they are only working while you are taking them – and that they will only mask the symptoms. They will not treat the reason why your bowel is going into spasm or giving you constipation or diarrhoea, and it is important to treat the cause otherwise you will have to take these drugs for life.

The next recommendation by NICE is that if the antispasmodic and either the laxatives or anti-diarrhoeal drugs do not work well enough, then you should be moved on to other medication, including tricyclic antidepressants (TCAs), followed by selective serotonin reuptake inhibitors (SSRIs) if these do not work.

ANTIDEPRESSANTS

It is thought that up to 95 per cent of your body's serotonin is located in your bowel. Antidepressants such as Prozac are designed to work by keeping serotonin levels in the brain high. In your digestive system, serotonin is released when food is in your intestines to make your gut contract around the food. If your digestive system is not happy with the food, for example it perceives it to be an irritant or 'off', it can release more serotonin to make the gut move faster, which gives you diarrhoea to clear out the food more quickly. And of course this involves more contractions of the bowel to move the food along faster and can result in pain and cramping. There is good evidence that antidepressants do work for IBS as the aim of using them is to change the way the muscles in your gut react and reduce the nerve response in your gut so that your brain registers less pain.[8] However, doctors can be reluctant to prescribe antidepressants for IBS because depression is not actually the main symptom being treated in this instance.[9]

The main antidepressants used for IBS are the TCAs and the SSRIs.

TRICYCLIC ANTIDEPRESSANTS (TCAS)

The once commonly prescribed TCAs for IBS are imipramine and amitriptyline. Low doses are given so that they work just on the bowel rather than on the mind.

Side effects can include dry mouth, blurred vision, drowsiness and constipation, so again this is a medication that could make your IBS symptoms worse if one of your main symptoms is constipation.

SELECTIVE SEROTONIN REUPTAKE INHIBITORS (SSRI)

The most well known SSRI is Prozac (fluoxetine) but with IBS other kinds are used. One called citalopram has been shown to help with abdominal pain and bloating but does not change the stool pattern so constipation or diarrhoea stays the same.[10]

Side effects can include headaches, nausea, insomnia and sexual problems.

SEROTONIN RECEPTOR MEDICATIONS

There is another group of medications which have an affect on serotonin. One in particular has been found to be helpful for women who experience more of the constipated kind of IBS. It does not seem to work for women who have the diarrhoea type or for men.

The medication is called tegaserod and is known as a selective 5-HT4 receptor agonist. It works by improving the movement of the gut, which helps with increasing bowel frequency, softening the stools and it also reduces sensitivity to pain within the gut.[11] This drug is available in most countries including the US but not in the UK and side effects can include diarrhoea, headache or joint pain. A rare side effect is a serious intestinal problem called ischemic colitis.

OVER-THE-COUNTER MEDICATIONS

Some medications that you can buy at the chemist or pharmacy without a prescription can be used to help with IBS symptoms. Some of them are over the counter versions of the prescription ones.

- **Antispasmodic medication** – mebeverine (see page 36) is available as an over-the-counter version known as Colofac.
- **Laxatives** – a number of laxatives are available to buy over the counter without a prescription and these incluce the bulking laxatives containing fibre such as Fybogel and Normacol. Osmotic laxatives such as movicol are also availble over the counter. The stimulant laxatives, which are best avoided with IBS, are also available without a prescription and include Senokot and Dulcolax.
- **Anti-diarrhoeal** – loperamide (commonly known as Immodium) can be bought directly from a chemist or pharmacy and helps by slowing down the movement of the stools, making them harder. But if you suspect that the diarrhoea has been caused by a bout of food poisoning then your body is giving you loose stools to try and expel the bug from your body, which is what you want to happen. My suggestion is to wait

a couple of days to see if the diarrhoea corrects itself, if you think it was caused by food. If it doesn't clear up, then see your doctor, as you may need prescription medication.

- **Painkillers** – you may be using painkillers to lessen the discomfort, but if you use ones like ibuprofen, which are classed as non-steroidal anti-inflammatories (NSAIDs) ,you could be making your symptoms worse as they will increase the risk of Leaky Gut (see page 50). If you have to use a painkiller, paracetamol would be a better choice.

As you can see, the medications used to treat IBS carry numerous side effects and if not managed properly can actually increase the symptoms you are trying to eliminate, or can cause you to swing between being constipated and having diarrhoea or vice versa. And I know from seeing patients in the clinic that you don't want to end up being on medication for the rest of your life or indeed have to take an extra drug to reduce the side effects of the first.

Medication can be very helpful in alleviating acute symptoms but will do little to tackle the root cause of the IBS. So I would encourage you to always feel what is right for your body. In the rest of the book I will be giving you all the very best natural ways to calm the irritation that is going in your bowels. There is research that acknowledges the drug-only approach has its limitations.[12] My approach will look at you as a whole person, not just what is going on in your bowels, because everything in your body is connected and I know from experience that this integrated way of approaching and then treating IBS is very successful.

CHAPTER 4

NUTRITIONAL TESTS

I outlined the diagnosis tests that you would expect to have investigated in Chapter 2. There are in addition a number of nutritional tests that have been developed that can add much clearer detail to an initial diagnosis of IBS. These tests can help determine the original cause in some cases and help you focus on what foods you should and should not be eating. We eat so many foods combined together each day that it makes teasing out the problem-causing foods very difficult, so a test for food allergies or sensitivities, for example, can be a good starting point.

This may seem like a lot of tests, but I want to show what is available to help you narrow down the possible causes and also to help you know what to eat and equip you with a plan of action.

TESTS TO ESTABLISH THE CAUSE OF IBS

FOOD ALLERGIES AND INTOLERANCES

Wouldn't it be wonderful if you could do a simple test that showed you what you should and shouldn't eat to help control your symptoms? The debate that surrounds testing for food allergies or intolerances for IBS is an interesting one and I will cover some of the issues on page 48.

But first of all it might be helpful to explain the difference between a food allergy and a food intolerance. Although people use the words interchangeably there is a major difference between the two.

Food Allergy

The word allergy is derived from Greek, with 'allos' meaning 'different' and 'ergos' meaning 'action'. This aptly describes what happens when we have an allergy: when something foreign enters your body, your body has to take action by responding differently to that alien substance. The earliest definition of 'allergy' was an 'inappropriate response by the body to a perfectly harmless substance'. But nowadays it is defined as a specific response by the immune system to a substance (inhaled, touched or eaten) that it mistakenly identifies as harmful. Well-known examples would be very severe reactions to peanuts or shellfish, where the response is immediate, no matter how much of the food has been eaten, and symptoms can include difficulty breathing, rashes, swelling, runny nose and possible anaphylactic shock, which can be fatal.

The allergy triggers the release of IgE antibodies, which attach to 'mast' cells and cause the release of histamine, the chemical which causes a contraction of the muscles around the air passages (an attack of breathlessness or asthma), local swelling and skin irritation, and, if the attack is serious enough, a drop in blood pressure.

This type of allergy can be tested by looking at the levels of IgE antibodies in a blood sample. A skin-prick test can also be used where small amounts of the allergens are tested on the arm or the back; a positive reaction would be shown by a hive or weal on the skin. Skin testing can be risky if you are suspected of having an allergy to a severe response-food, such as peanuts, for example, so a blood test may be preferred. The gold standard for diagnosing a food allergy, however, is oral food challenging, where someone is given a suspect food and the reaction is monitored. This is considered the best method, but needs to be done under medical supervision in a clinical setting.[1]

Food Intolerances

There is another type of reaction to food called food intolerances and it is also known as food sensitivity or non-allergic hypersensitivity. With these reactions there can be a delay in the onset of the symptoms (from four to seventy-two hours), and the foods are often eaten in larger amounts and more frequently. Symptoms can be varied, from bloating, diarrhoea, constipation and flatulence to lethargy, arthritis, fatigue, skin rashes, eczema, joint and muscle pains, recurrent infections, anxiety, depression, insomnia, irritability, water retention, headaches, migraines and generally feeling unwell.

This type of reaction can be broken down into three different types:

- Lack of an enzyme
- Chemical reaction
- Raised IgG antibodies

Lack of an Enzyme

People with this type of food intolerance don't produce a particular enzyme that helps them break down a certain food. The most common one is lactose intolerance. Lactose is a sugar which is found in milk (it is also called milk sugar) and you have to have the enzyme lactase in your body in order to break down the lactose, which otherwise can cause common IBS symptoms as it sits fermenting in the gut causing pain, gas and bloating. Testing for lactose intolerance can be done with a hydrogen breath test because when lactose ferments in the gut it produces hydrogen which can be measured in the breath.

Chemical Reactions

This is where the reaction is caused by a chemical within the food rather than you lacking an enzyme. One of the most common food intolerances of this kind is caused by chemicals called amines.

Contained in foods like cheese, citrus fruits, red wine, chocolate and coffee, amines can trigger migraines in those who are sensitive to these substances by causing blood vessels to expand. Chemical reactions to foods are usually picked up by doing an elimination diet and seeing if symptoms improve and then introducing the foods again to see of the symptoms return.

Some people may react to chemicals that have been added to foods rather than those that are naturally occurring. Examples of these additives include MSG, a flavouring, and sodium benzoate, a preservative. Symptoms can include abdominal pain, diarrhoea and skin reactions. You may find that you can 'get away' with a small amount of the chemical but when you have too much it causes a reaction.

MSG can occur naturally in some foods including, cheeses, stock cubes, meat extracts, mushrooms and yeast extracts. But I would be more careful when the MSG is added to the food as a flavour enhancer as the levels can be much higher. The other additives to watch out for are benzoates, nitrates, sulphites, tartrazine, Sunset Yellow and aspartame. You can read the labels to see whether the foods you are buying contain these additives because food companies have to list them in the ingredients if they use them.

- **Benzoates** – used as a preservative and often found in canned drinks, desserts and juices such as aloe vera. They may also be used in cosmetics and toiletries under the name 'parabens' and there are concerns they may increase oestrogen levels, disrupting your body's natural hormone balance.
- **Nitrates** – these are often found in processed meats such as bacon and salami to give the meat a pink colour and also in some cheeses, such as Edam. The problem is that the nitrates can form nitrites – which are known to form cancer-causing substances – when eaten. They can also form nitrites before

you eat them, due to the cooking process, and the higher the temperature the worse the problem, for example when barbecuing processed meats such as sausages.

- **Sulphites** – often found in juices and especially in wines. These can be used to preserve dried fruit so avoid those packets of dried fruit which have sulphur dioxide on the label (they are often used in dried apricots to prevent them going brown, for example).
- **Tartrazine** – a synthetic dye made from coal tar that gives food a yellow colour. It is found in so many different foods and drinks that you will have to read the labels. It can also be found in some medications.
- **Sunset Yellow** – this colouring is manufactured from petroleum and is found in many different foods – most often in orange squash to give a bright yellow colour.
- **Aspartame** – this is an artificial sweetener used in many foods and drinks and often in sports or diet drinks, where the manufacturer is aiming to reduce or eliminate added sugar from the product.

My advice is to become a label reader. You only have to do it for a short while until you get to know the brands and products that are additive-free. I have been working in the nutrition field for over thirty years and it is much easier now to buy 'clean' foods and drinks than it ever was before. If in doubt don't buy the product, because there is sure to be another brand without the additives. (See the box 'Nasties' in Your Food and Drinks on page 118 for more information about additives.)

Raised IgG Antibodies

The third type of food intolerance reaction is the production of IgG antibodies. This is a controversial area in testing for food intolerances and I will mention it here in some detail because there is so much confusion around allergy and intolerance testing. The medical profession says that there is only one kind of food allergy and that it is when IgE antibodies are raised – all the rest are food intolerances (see page 45). And yet many people will send off for food sensitivity blood testing kits from the web that measure IgG antibodies rather than IgE. What are they really measuring and are they worth it?

On the one hand we have the medical allergists who say that a healthy immune system is supposed to make IgG antibodies in response to foreign substances (proteins), and a positive IgG test to a food is therefore a sign of a normal immune system rather than a reaction to a particular food. As one study commented about IgG antibodies, 'These lack scientific rationale, standardization and reproducibility. There have been no well-designed studies to support these tests and in fact, several authors have disproved their utility.'[2]

However, a separate study commented that IgG testing for food intolerance 'showed promise with clinically meaningful results. It has been proven useful as a guide for elimination diets with clinical impact for a variety of diseases.'[3]

Confused? I don't blame you. If the medical and scientific experts can't agree amongst themselves then it makes it even harder for you to know what is useful as a test for foods you may be reacting to.

In my clinical experience the two main culprits of food intolerance are dairy and wheat, which also tend to have the highest levels of IgG when tested. So I believe it is worth excluding these first, and monitoring your symptoms. In the next chapter I will give you a seven-day Diet Plan to get you started and help you listen to your body, as it really is the best way to finding those foods that are symptom triggers for you.

A worrying trend I have seen is that when people eliminate all the foods that they show a reaction to from the IgG antibodies blood test

BIORESONANCE MACHINES AND MUSCLE TESTING

There are other ways of testing for food and substance allergies or intolerances that use bioresonance machines (or electrodermal testing) and muscle testing but I have reservations about their effectiveness.

A bioresonance machine is a type of non-invasive scanning machine that often uses one or more acupuncture points while a person is asked to hold different foods and substances. The machine shows what may or may not cause an imbalance for that person.

Muscle testing (sometimes called applied kinesiology) is done without a machine. You are asked to hold your arm out to the side while the practitioner presses down on it to see how you resist the pressure. You are then given a food or substance to hold and the same amount of pressure is applied. It is thought that if you can resist the pressure then the food or substance is fine for you but if your arm collapses then it is a food or substance you should avoid.

In my opinion, these kinds of food allergy or intolerance tests are not objective enough because they depend on the skill and often interpretation and judgement of the practitioner. I think it is far preferable to send a blood sample to a laboratory to get an objective measurement that can't be influenced.

results, their symptoms can initially get better but gradually they often return. When they repeat the blood test later on, they then react to a different list of foods. So over time their diet becomes more and more restricted. This leads me to think that we are not actually treating the cause of the problem and rather than an intolerance to those foods, the IgG antibodies could be an indicator of something else.

We do know that high levels of IgG antibodies are associated with inflammation and inflammatory substances are produced in the gut as a response to the IgG antibodies.[4] This is why scientists are now suggesting that when you have IBS there is 'mini-inflammation' going on in the bowel which can make you much more sensitive to different foods and increase levels of pain and spasms.[5] The inflammation also damages the wall of your intestines. This damage causes 'leaky gut' where the intestines can't prevent the 'leakage' of large particles through the intestinal wall into general blood circulation. Food molecules can escape into the blood stream, which then sets up an immune response by causing the body to treat these food particles as foreign substances and attack them. This is how you can react to foods that previously gave you no problems at all. So when you test for IgG antibodies and they come back high I think that the test is often showing that you have a leaky gut (also called Intestinal Permeability).

LEAKY GUT (INTESTINAL PERMEABILITY)

Your gut should act as a barrier to prevent toxins and large molecules escaping into your bloodstream. When the gut becomes 'leaky' it loses the ability to act as a barrier and this increased permeability is associated with reacting inappropriately to some foods but also to autoimmune diseases, skin problems and inflammation in general, especially in the joints. Having a gut that is too permeable allows food particles to escape through your gut wall and sets up an immune reaction, making you react negatively to certain foods, but this is not a true food allergy.

Testing for leaky gut is particularly important if you have mainly the diarrhoea type of IBS symptoms because you are at an increased risk of having leaky gut. Research has shown that having increased permeability increases your sensitivity to pain in the gut and leads to more severe IBS symptoms.[6]

The test is simple and comprises a non-invasive urine test with the samples collected at home. Two urine samples are needed. The first is a pre-test sample to give a baseline reading and the second urine sample is collected six hours after drinking a special liquid which contains two marker molecules. When the samples are analysed, the amount of these marker molecules detected in the laboratory give a strong indication as to how 'leaky' your gut is.

If the test shows you have a leaky gut you will be given recommend-ations as to how to heal it back up again using natural remedies. You can then re-test the leaky gut in three months time to make sure that it is back to normal. The diet and nutrition recommendations in this book will go a long way to help with leaky gut. It is really important therefore to identify the foods which trigger your IBS symptoms and exclude those while your gut heals. I have also included a note on supplements for leaky gut on page 134.

Note: The liquid used to ascertain whether you have a leaky gut contains lactulose and mannitol and it is recommended that you do not do this test if you already know you react to sorbitol, xylitol or lactulose, or if you are already on a lactose-free diet.

CANDIDA ANTIBODY TEST

An overgrowth of candida (candiasis) can give you many IBS symptoms such as bloating, diarrhoea and constipation as well as headaches, fatigue and muscle aches. Years ago there was a trend for many patients I saw in the clinic to follow an anti-candida diet. It can be very effective, but this kind of diet is also extremely restrictive and involves removing foods and drinks that increase the growth of yeast, such as those that contain added sugar or yeasts, fermented prod-ucts like alcohol, and certain fruits. For this reason it is important to establish whether you do truly have a problem with candida before embarking on such a strict diet and I would recommend being tested under the supervision of a nutritionist. Please see the contact details for my clinic, where we offer both testing and treatment, on page 207. Getting candida under control doesn't just require you to change what you eat; you also have to replenish your gut bacteria and take certain supplements to eliminate the overgrowth.

There is a simple saliva test which checks for an overgrowth of candida. You collect a sample of saliva in the container supplied and then post it back to the laboratory. If you have a candida overgrowth then candida antibodies will be present in your saliva, which indicates that your body is trying to fight the yeast infection. You will then be given recommendations as to how to change your diet, what to take to replenish beneficial bacteria and how to eliminate the candida overgrowth.

SECRETORY IGA

This is also a saliva test like the candida antibody test and a sample can be collected at home. Secretory IgA is your first line of defence against bacteria, yeasts and problem foods. The problem is if you have a deficiency of Secretory IgA then you do not have the ability to fight off infections, especially in the gut. If you are deficient then a supplement of Saccharomyces boulardii may be helpful as it increases the levels of this antibody (see page 135).

CASE STUDY: ANGELA

Angela, sixty-two, came to one of my clinics with general digestive problems including constipation, flatulence and bloating and gastritis (an inflammation of the stomach which is different to IBS). She had never been referred for any medical tests, but instead had been given a proton pump inhibitor (a drug that reduces the secretion of stomach acid in order to try and reduce the inflammation) for the gastritis. This was slowly becoming ineffective and she had got to the point where she felt that every time she ate it bloated her stomach.

My nutritionist went through a detailed questionnaire with her which revealed there was a lot of stress in Angela's life that she really felt exacerbated her IBS. She also had a history of repeated antibiotic use. She was advised to perform a stool analysis to help identify what was happening at a deeper level. Because Angela had never done any tests she was enthusiastic to get on with the stool analysis to see if it would shed some light as to why she has been suffering.

In the meantime she was advised to follow a gluten-free diet, using more brown rice, buckwheat and quinoa, and to cut out caffeine, which could be irritating her gut. She was sent away with a food diary to complete daily and some gentle supplements including aloe vera, magnesium and slippery elm. The supplement programme had to be carefully put together because certain digestive supplements are not suitable when someone has gastritis.

Angela came back for her follow-up consultation once her test results were back and to her surprise (because this had never been picked up) it showed very low beneficial bacteria, a yeast infection and very low Secretory IgA (SIgA). SIgA is secreted by the mucosal tissue in the gut and represents the first line of defence, acting as an immune barrier. These low levels would make her more susceptible to food sensitivity and invasion of bacteria and yeast.

After explaining the findings of the stool test in detail, the nutritionist modified Angela's supplement programme to include a good probiotic and Saccharomyces boulardii, which specifically 'feeds' the SIgA. She continued with the aloe vera and slippery elm because these already, together with the Diet Plan, were making such a difference.

After three months Angela was pretty much symptom-free with occasional relapses but when these did occur, she knew it was either due to stress or not being consistent with her diet and supplements. In the long term Angela may be able to tolerate a wider range of foods and certainly reduce the supplements with the support of her nutritionist.

HELICOBACTER PYLORI (H PYLORI)

Checking for H pylori is useful if you are getting symptoms that are concentrated more in the upper part of your digestive tract such as heartburn (acid reflux), indigestion that occurs two to three hours after eating or during the night, nausea and vomiting. H pylori is thought to be the only bacteria that can survive the strong acid in your stomach. It is now known that H pylori is the major cause of gastric, duodenal ulcers and gastritis (inflammation of the lining of the stomach).

It is better to do a breath test to check for H pylori than a blood test as the latter is looking for an antibody to those bacteria. If you have had H pylori in the past, then you will have produced an antibody to it and a blood test may show a positive result even though you may not have an active present infection. The test would just be reflecting a past immune system response.

A breath test is much more accurate because it measures ammonia and carbon dioxide, the substances that are released when there is an active H pylori infection. The test requires you to give two breath samples, thirty minutes apart, after a six hour fast (preferably overnight). Samples can be collected at home and then sent back to the laboratory in the packaging provided. If you are diagnosed with H pylori infection then your doctor will give you treatment to eradicate it.

SMALL INTESTINAL BACTERIAL OVERGROWTH (SIBO)

It is now thought that many of the symptoms of IBS are due to bacteria overgrowth in the small intestine (SIBO). As you know, the small intestine's role is mainly to digest and absorb your food and then any food that has not been digested and absorbed is passed into the large intestines where water is absorbed from the waste and then moved along to be excreted. The majority of the bacteria in the gut are actually in the large intestines and these bacteria also help in the digestive process by feeding off the undigested food. These bacteria produce valuable substances, such as fatty acids, but also gas through fermentation.

But some people actually have a very large number of organisms in the small intestines which means that foods gets fermented there instead of being digested. And the kind of bacteria in the small intestines is similar to what would be normally found in the large intestines.

Symptoms are often similar to those associated with IBS, including excess gas, abdominal pain and bloating, and often diarrhoea. The test for SIBO involves swallowing lactulose and then collecting breath samples every twenty minutes for three hours. The presence of SIBO is assessed by measuring hydrogen and methane in the breath.

This means that if the test shows you are positive for SIBO then you *can* be treated with probiotics and usually a short term antibiotic. And in some ways getting a positive test for SIBO is good news because research suggests that symptoms which are being labelled as IBS are actually SIBO so you now have a cause and something can be done about it, because you can be given medication to treat it.[7]

STOOL TEST

I think a stool test can be extremely useful in trying to determine the cause of IBS because it is well known that having a bout of food poisoning can leave you twice as likely to develop IBS and, in my experience, that 'bug' may still be there causing you symptoms.[8]

The stool test I use in the clinic gives you much more information than just checking for bugs or parasites. It actually assesses how well you can digest and absorb your food, especially your ability to absorb fats, which are often a trigger for IBS symptoms. This stool test also gives a measure of how much of the beneficial bacteria, like lactobacillus and bifidobacterium, you have in your gut. When you are checking for parasites, it is important that you give three stool samples, not just one, because the parasite may not be picked up on only one sample.

ADRENAL STRESS TEST

If your IBS or general digestive symptoms seem to reduce when you are on holiday and feeling relaxed then a big part of the problem might be your stress levels. There is now a simple laboratory test that measures your levels of cortisol, the main indicator of stress, using samples of saliva.

Both adrenaline and cortisol are your 'stress' hormones but adrenaline is so short lived in the body that it is almost impossible to test for it, but we can measure the other stress hormone, cortisol. This test measures your levels of cortisol from four saliva samples given at different times of the day. It is important not to test at just one time of day because cortisol has a circadian or 'daily' rhythm and should be at its highest in the morning and then reduce throughout the day until it is at its lowest level at night before you go to bed.

The test not only measures cortisol but also another adrenal hormone, DHEA (dehydroepiandrosterone), which is the hormone that works to balance many of the negative effects of cortisol and helps you cope with stress.

Stress is often a part of the IBS puzzle, even if it is not the main culprit. It is so easy to get caught up in a cycle of anxiety about food that worsens the symptoms, which in turn makes you more stressed than ever. Chapter 7 explores the many ways we can help to maintain healthy stress levels, from relaxation techniques to foods and supplements that help support the adrenals and keep the body relaxed.

For more information on obtaining this test, see Useful Resources on page 207.

TESTS TO ESTABLISH WHAT FOODS YOU CAN AND CANNOT EAT

We have now covered the tests that can help narrow down the cause of your IBS symptoms so let us have a look at those tests that can help you know what you should be eating.

COELIAC DISEASE

Coeliac disease is an immune response to the protein gluten, which is contained in certain grains and ends up damaging the lining of the small intestines. It is not strictly speaking an allergy to gluten or wheat but an autoimmune disease in which the gluten in the grain (wheat, barley and rye) triggers the immune system to produce antibodies that, over time, damage the lining of the small intestines by flattening down the villi in the small intestines, making it harder for the body to absorb nutrients from food.

Symptoms of coeliac disease can include diarrhoea, abdominal pain, mouth ulcers, anaemia, weight loss and skin problems such as psoriasis, but not everyone gets the same symptoms. You should have been tested for coeliac disease as part of your IBS screening in the first place, but if you haven't it is important that you get this done. Recent research in 2011 suggested that everyone suffering with IBS should be routinely tested for coeliac disease because it is a common finding.[9]

The test for coeliac disease is straightforward – it is a simple blood test which checks for antibodies to gluten and also tissue transglutam-inase and endomysial antibodies. Having a positive result overall on these markers on the blood test gives an accuracy of 99 per cent that you have coeliac disease and it is not always necessary nowadays to go on to have a small intestine biopsy to confirm the diagnosis. If you think you might have coeliac disease you need to be tested before you start eliminating gluten from your diet, otherwise the test can give a false negative reading because your gluten-free diet will stop your body producing the antibodies that are picked up on the blood test.

If you are coeliac then you will need to eliminate gluten from your diet (see page 68).

GLUTEN SENSITIVITY

Over the last few years there has been recognition that a person can be sensitive to gluten but not have full-blown coeliac disease. So you might have symptoms that are similar to those experienced in coeliac disease but a blood test will be negative for antibodies and you won't have damage to the small intestines. When this is the case you might still benefit greatly from a gluten-free diet (see page 68) and see dramatic improvements in your IBS symptoms and your sense of health and wellbeing in general.[10] Symptoms of gluten sensitivity can include not only gastrointestinal ones such as bloating, abdominal pain or discomfort, diarrhoea, constipation but also tiredness, lethargy, migraines, headaches and joint pains. Recent research suggests that gluten sensitivity is extremely common and could affect up to 10 per cent of people compared to 1 per cent for coeliac disease.[11]

If you undergo a full blood test for coeliac disease, including all the markers mentioned on page 57, then it is possible to differentiate between having coeliac disease and being gluten sensitive, depending on which markers are positive and which are negative.

WHEAT ALLERGY

I will mention wheat allergy briefly just to make clear the difference between a wheat allergy, coeliac disease and gluten sensitivity.

A wheat allergy is the type of allergy mentioned on page 44, where you would have an IgE antibody reaction to one of the proteins in wheat, as measured on a blood test. Symptoms can include nausea, bloating, hives and also breathing difficulties. And like other IgE reactions to other foods, such as peanuts and shellfish, it can cause a life-threatening anaphylactic allergic response.

When a person has a wheat allergy they only have to eliminate wheat from their diet, not other grains such as rye and barley (which a coeliac would have to eliminate).

LACTOSE INTOLERANCE TEST

It is now thought that up to 27 per cent of IBS sufferers might also be lactose intolerant. Dairy products contain lactose, which is milk sugar, and for it to be absorbed into the bloodstream from your gut it has to be broken down into two other sugars, glucose and galactose, by an enzyme called lactase. If someone does not have enough of this enzyme lactase then the lactose remains undigested in the gut and ferments, giving symptoms such as diarrhoea, abdominal pain, gas and bloating, all typical IBS symptoms.

If you want to know whether you are lactose intolerant you need to take a hydrogen breath test. When lactose ferments in the gut it produces hydrogen so when you breathe out it can be measured. You are given a dose of pure lactose and then readings of hydrogen are taken from your breath over a number of minutes. If the hydrogen level is high then it would indicate you are lactose intolerant.

What is particularly of note is that removing milk seems to help IBS sufferers *whether they are lactose intolerant or not*, so it may not be just that the lactose in the milk is the culprit but that there are other factors in dairy that upset IBS sufferers (see page 69).[12]

If there is a positive reaction to the test, then it would be worth eliminating foods containing lactose to see if this makes a difference. If it doesn't, then it may be a bacterial overgrowth, which causes fermentation symptoms that can trigger a positive result.[13]. The test for bacterial overgrowth is mentioned on page 55. A course of antibiotics (also using probiotics to offset the negative effects of the antibiotics) may be a useful treatment for some people with bacterial overgrowth.[14]

FRUCTOSE INTOLERANCE TEST

Fructose is the sugar found in fruit but is also used as a sweetener in many products in the form of fructose corn syrup. Fructose intolerance is thought to be the cause of many of the symptoms found in IBS.[15] This has led to the development of the FODMAP diet (see page 108), which restricts foods containing fructose and polyols (another sugar) as well as those which are fermentable (like lentils and wheat) or that contain lactose. This restrictive diet is really only recommended if you have tried excluding individual food groups to no avail (see Chapter 5).

A sample of fructose in water is given for the test and samples are collected every hour for three hours. An increase in hydrogen would indicate fructose intolerance.

These nutrition tests can be very helpful in narrowing down the possible causes and triggers of your IBS symptoms. If you have a sense, for example, that you may be experiencing candidiasis (an overgrowth of candida) symptoms you can order a quick test rather than go headlong into the anti-candida diet, which is extremely restrictive and takes a serious commitment. If you did receive a positive result for a test, you would be able to focus on more specific ways to help your own case of IBS, especially as you begin to focus on healing your IBS through your diet, which I will guide you through step by step in the next chapter.

Many of these tests can be organized by post from www.natural-healthpractice.com, which is helpful if you cannot get into one of my clinics. See Useful Resources on page 208 for more details.

PART TWO

NATURAL
SOLUTIONS
TO IBS

CHAPTER 5

EATING TO BEAT IBS

For me this is the most important chapter in the book because the majority of people with IBS feel their symptoms are worsened by certain foods.[1] I want to encourage you to think that food can be of great benefit to the healing process and to convince you that there are foods which can help soothe and calm your system, rather than be a source of irritation. It can be easy to fall into having very negative thoughts about all food if you are suffering from IBS. Rather than associating food with health and vitality, you may begin to associate it with pain and discomfort. It is my aim to help you see that in addition to learning to recognize potential food triggers, you will also discover lots of delicious and healing alternatives too.

Everyone is different and your dietary triggers may be different from those of someone else with IBS; sometimes it is not only the food itself but the timing of when you eat or even the amount. And it can also make a big difference if you are feeling stressed on the day that you eat a particular food (see Chapter 7 on stress).

I don't want you to waste time, or indeed feel miserable, on an overly restricted diet if it's not right for you, so I would suggest you follow this chapter one step at a time, and do the easiest dietary suggestions first because if they work for you first time then wonderful

– you won't need to do anything more restrictive or complicated. If they don't, then you can move on to the next step.

First I will cover exclusion diets and the different foods you can exclude to see if they have an effect on your symptoms. This is particularly good if you already have an idea of the specific foods that might be triggering your IBS. If, however, you really are in the dark and need a place to start, I recommend you go straight on to my Diet Plan. This excludes the most common problem IBS foods and offers a complete meal plan full of IBS-friendly ingredients to help your digestive system heal. If after the Diet Plan or your own exclusion plan you still suffer from IBS symptoms, I suggest you go on to the much more restrictive FODMAP diet.

You may have decided to take one or more of the nutrition tests available, as outlined in the previous chapter, and so maybe you now know that you have a lactose intolerance or perhaps you need to take care of your stress levels. The Diet Plan I recommend in this chapter is designed to be a healthy start for the majority of the types of IBS I see in my clinic. In essence, it is a healthy diet that makes things much easier on your gut and gives it a chance to heal and strengthen so that you can then begin to add back in a wider variety of foods over time. And it is so important to do that. If you restrict yourself to a very small number of foods for a long time then often your gut will begin to struggle with these too. So once you begin to feel better and more confident then I hope you will enjoy gradually trying new foods once again and live an IBS-free life.

So I want you to be reassured that many of these dietary changes are not for ever; the idea is to remove foods that are causing you a problem now and keep assessing the situation. Give your gut a rest, let it calm down and get back to health.

EXCLUSION DIET

Often the first dietary suggestion is to try a so-called exclusion (also called an elimination) diet where certain foods and food groups are eliminated for about two weeks. Success rates from exclusion diets can range from 15 to 71 per cent so it really depends on the individual. They do take quite a bit of commitment but if you are able to discover specific foods that are triggering your symptoms this kind of diet can be well worth it in the long run.[2]

Exclusion diets can exclude a number of different foods, the main ones being gluten, wheat (as it is not always the gluten which is the culprit), dairy, processed meats, potatoes, citrus fruits, caffeinated drinks and alcohol. Less common foods that may also trigger symptoms include fermentable foods like legumes (beans, lentils, etc.), tomatoes, onions, peppers, broccoli, cabbage and cucumber (for some, just the skin seems to cause indigestion). Also, high-fat, greasy or spicy foods can be a problem, as can artificial sweeteners.

There is no one universally advised exclusion diet and so it is often more of a case of trial and error for the individual. However, I have some guidelines that I give to patients that can really help to identify any specific food triggers sooner rather than later:

- Keep a food and symptom diary throughout so that you can detect any pattern to your symptoms. You should keep an eye out for foods that trigger symptoms, but you may also discover that there are certain times of the day which are worse or that your symptoms are linked to regularly stressful aspects of your week (see Chapter 7).
- I recommend to patients that they try excluding **wheat and dairy foods** first for two weeks. Keep a careful note of your symptoms and if they have gone after two weeks, introduce

one of these foods groups back in to your diet gradually over two days to see if you get a flare up of symptoms or not. If not, then bring the other foods back in.

You can follow this formula for any number of foods but keep in mind it does take two weeks of exclusion before you can reintroduce the food to test if it is a trigger. It is also important to leave two days in between testing foods because the reaction can often be slower than you think as the food passes through the digestive system.

I'll now go into more detail about excluding wheat (and gluten in wheat) and dairy from your diet.

EXCLUDING WHEAT AND DAIRY

Why would wheat and dairy cause the biggest problems? It might seem unfair that the foods we think of as such core staples in our diet are often the likeliest IBS triggers. But it is because we eat such large quantities of these foods relative to everything else in our daily diet that explains why we can become so sensitive to them.

Apart from the obvious sources of wheat (bread, pasta, biscuits and cakes) and dairy (milk, cheese and yoghurt) many different types of food can contain them. Wheat is often found in:

- Sausages – used as a filler
- Sauces – used as a thickener
- Soups
- Gravy and stock cubes
- Soy sauce

Dairy foods can also be found in:

- Breakfast cereals
- Cereal bars

- Processed meats
- Some breads

It is interesting that if we look back in time, grains like wheat and also dairy were very infrequently eaten by people before agriculture was introduced about 10,000 years ago.[3] As humans we have been on the earth for around 200,000 years, which makes grains and dairy relatively 'new' foods. Our digestive systems would have had to try to adapt to them and it is possible that certain people may have adapted better than others.

Fibre

Over the years there has been a lot of discussion about how much fibre you should eat if you suffer from IBS; sometimes high fibre has been suggested and other times low fibre. It seems much clearer now that it is not fibre per se that may be the problem but the *type* of fibre.

There are two forms of fibre, soluble (which dissolves in water) and insoluble (which doesn't). Soluble fibre is found in oats, barley, peas, flaxseed (linseed) and some fruits and vegetables. It turns to a gel during digestion and can help with both constipation and diarrhoea. With diarrhoea, the soluble fibre acts as a bulking agent to make the stool more formed, and with constipation it helps make the stool softer and wetter so that it passes out more easily and comfortably.

Insoluble fibre is found in wheat and particularly bran. It holds on to water and can have a greater laxative effect, so it's not good if your IBS symptom is predominantly diarrhoea rather than constipation. Insoluble fibre is often known as roughage because it can be pretty 'rough' on the digestive system. And the consensus seems to be that insoluble fibre can make the IBS symptoms worse.[4] It makes sense, therefore, to exclude wheat and bran to avoid the insoluble fibre they contain.

Be aware that a number of foods will contain both soluble and insoluble fibre, such as fruits and vegetables in which the insoluble fibre is mainly in the skin.

Gluten

Sometimes IBS sufferers are advised to go for white bread and pasta as wholewheat can cause more problems because of the insoluble fibre in the whole grain (see above). However, I don't think eating a refined food, stripped of all its goodness, is good for your health. And more often than not, the real culprit is the amount of gluten found in wheat, which causes a problem whether you eat the whole or refined grain.

Gluten is a protein found naturally in the grain. Over years the gluten content of wheat has been altered to be increasingly high so that the grain does not fall apart as it goes through commercial bakery machines. Obviously, commercial bread is not made by hand and so the grain has to be robust enough to endure the factory process.

Gluten acts like glue; it is stretchy and sticky (think of how a mixture of flour and water is often used as a paste for gluing papier-mâché). The problem is that it has the same effect inside your body, making it hard to digest and also absorb nutrients. You may also suffer from symptoms such as abdominal pain, bloating and diarrhoea (sounds like IBS, doesn't it?) as well as other non-digestive related symptoms such as tiredness, headaches and joint pains.

Grains like rye and barley also contain some gluten, but in much smaller amounts than wheat, so you may find you are less sensitive to these alternative grains. Oats don't naturally contain gluten but they can often become contaminated with gluten during growing because the oats can be next to the wheat fields and can also be contaminated during the milling process. There are now gluten-free oats available but some people who react to gluten can also react to a protein in the oats called avenin, which is similar to gluten. You may need to exclude all grains for two weeks and then gradually reintroduce them to see which trigger symptoms and which you are able to eat without issue.

Spelt is another grain that contains gluten and is often called 'ancient wheat' because it is one of the original strains of wheat. The gluten in spelt is different from the gluten in wheat in that it is much easier to digest and a number of people who find wheat a problem can tolerate spelt. You use spelt in cooking in exactly the same way as wheat.

My suggestion is to first eliminate wheat and dairy (see below) and then if your symptoms are much improved, try experimenting with small amounts of spelt and see what happens. Quantity can make a big difference, so just have small amounts to start with, don't overload your body.

Dairy

Dairy products contain lactose, which is milk sugar, and for it to be absorbed into the bloodstream from your gut it has to be broken down by an enzyme called lactase into two other sugars, glucose and galactose. If someone does not have enough of the lactase enzyme then the lactose remains undigested in the gut and ferments, giving symptoms such as diarrhoea, abdominal pain, gas and bloating – all typical IBS symptoms.

We know that about 15 per cent of Caucasians and 70–90 per cent of Asians, Black Africans and American Indians are lactose intolerant because they stop producing the milk-digesting enzyme lactase when they enter adulthood. We are the only animal to drink milk beyond the weaning stage; plus we drink the milk of other animals. There are some cultures in which dairy and wheat are eaten very infrequently, such as most Asian cultures, where rice is more predominant. In these Eastern cultures the prevalence of IBS has always been low but with the emerging new economies and the introduction of more Western-style food, IBS levels are increasing.[5]

Lactose is contained in most dairy products including milk, ice cream and soft cheeses. The higher the fat content of the dairy food, the lower the amount of lactose, so full-fat milk will contain less lactose than skimmed.

Many traditional cultures around the world do include dairy in their diet but have it fermented in some way, for example yoghurt and kefir. Yoghurt does contain lactose but the beneficial bacteria seem to help break it down and so many people can tolerate natural yoghurt without any problem. Also, hard cheeses and butter have very low levels of lactose and some, none at all. The problem is that you cannot tell the lactose content from the label on the food and so checking your own responses is the best way to be sure.

It is now thought that up to 27 per cent of IBS sufferers can be lactose intolerant but what is particularly interesting is that removing dairy seems to help IBS sufferers whether they are lactose intolerant or not, so it may not be just the lactose in the milk that is the culprit.[6] There are proteins in dairy foods such as whey and casein that can cause digestive upsets but new research suggests that the major problem may be the **fat** in the dairy foods.

Research with milk fat has shown that it upsets the delicate balance of bacteria within the gut and causes the proliferation of a microbe called Bilophila wadsworthia (B wadsworthia), which is found in inflammatory bowel diseases (bear in mind we know that those with IBS suffer from mini-inflammation). Milk fats are difficult to digest and the liver has to release a particular form of bile that is rich in sulphur to help break down these fats. But this microbe B wadsworthia thrives in a sulphur-rich environment, and the by-products of this microbe are classed as 'gut mucosal barrier breakers' because they can cause leaky gut, which can increase sensitivity to foods (see page 50).[7]

You can buy lactose-reduced milk in some supermarkets, or you can take the enzyme lactase to break down the lactose, either as a liquid supplement to add to milk or as a food supplement half an hour before having dairy food.

I have been working in the nutrition field now for over thirty years and it used to be difficult to get non-dairy alternatives but nowadays you can buy rice, oat and nut milks in supermarkets. If you are worried about not getting enough calcium while you exclude dairy from your diet there are good non-dairy sources. An adult needs about 700mg of calcium a day and it is easy to make this up with the foods in the table below. I will also include information on how to supplement with calcium and other nutrients in Chapter 6.

NON-DAIRY SOURCES OF CALCIUM

Food (100g portion)		Calcium (mg)
Fish	Pilchards in tomato sauce	250
	Sardines in tomato sauce	430
	Sardines in oil	500
	Whitebait, fried	860
Vegetables	Curly kale, boiled	150
	Okra, stir-fried	220
	Spring greens, boiled	75
	Watercress	170
Pulses, beans and seeds	Baked beans	53
	Green/French beans	56
	Red kidney beans	71
	Sesame seeds	670
	Tahini (sesame paste)	680
	Tofu, steamed*	510

* Different products will vary considerably

NON-DAIRY SOURCES OF CALCIUM (cont.)

Food (100g portion)		Calcium (mg)
Fruit	Apricots, dried	73
	Currants	93
	Figs, dried	250
	Mixed peel	130
	Olives, in brine	61
	Orange	47

EXCLUDING OTHER FOODS

There are other food groups that may or may not be a culprit when it comes to triggering your IBS symptoms and after trying the wheat and dairy exclusion diet for two weeks you may want to look at these other foods. I will explore each of them here, and you may immediately recognize some which affect you or you might need to experiment to find those foods that are best to avoid while your gut is healing. Writing a food and mood diary is a very good way to track what you are eating and start to see patterns that connect individual foods or food groups with specific symptoms you experience. Write down everything you eat and drink for a week, and make a note of how you feel physically and mentally about one to two hours after having that food and drink. You might then start to see a pattern around certain foods that are affecting you.

Resistant Starch

As the name implies, resistant starch means that it resists digestion. It avoids getting digested in the small intestines and ends up fermenting in the large intestines. It is also called fermentable carbohydrate.

Normally, resistant starch is a good thing to include in your diet because these types of carbohydrate do not rapidly convert into glucose (sugar) and so they are low on the glycaemic index (GI). According to the World Health Organization, resistant starch is the only dietary constituent which shows a convincing protective effect against weight gain.[8] As it does not get converted to sugar quickly, it helps to control your blood sugar (glucose) levels,[9] and also helps to improve insulin sensitivity.[10]

But resistant starch may not be so helpful if you have IBS, as these foods can ferment in the digestive tract, causing bloating, abdominal discomfort, flatulence, trapped wind and diarrhoea.[11] The thing is that everyone has a different tolerance to these kinds of starches and some of you may find that they cause a lot of digestive discomfort while others may be able to tolerate them perfectly well.[12] It really is a case of trial and error, and the best way forward is to reduce resistant starches drastically, see what happens to your symptoms, then gradually try them one at a time and monitor the impact.

Foods that contain resistant starch include:

- Legumes (for example chickpeas, beans and lentils)
- Unripe fruit (for example green bananas)
- Wholegrains and seeds (rice, barley, pasta, oats and wheat)
- Cooked, cold food (potatoes, rice and pasta)

There are two forms of starch: amylose and amylopectin. Amylose is the most resistant because it is a tighter molecule and harder for your body to break down. Most starchy carbohydrates will contain a mixture of both amylose and amylopectin. But some, such as beans and peas, can contain more amylose and it is this that can give certain people more symptoms.

Legumes have a high content of resistant starch because they have thick cell walls, making it difficult for the digestive enzymes to break down the starch for digestion. Broccoli, cauliflower and cabbage may also cause excess wind. For some people these vegetables are not digested completely in the small intestines, maybe due to a lack of enzymes. It means that when they reach the large intestines, bacteria in that part of the gut can cause gas when breaking down those foods.

Cooking breaks down the cell walls of foods, making the starch more available for digestion and therefore less resistant. But cooking and then cooling food and eating it cold actually *increases* resistant starch content. For example, the starch is broken down when you cook potatoes, but when left to cool, starch that is formed by the cooling process becomes resistant to digestion. So if you have IBS and want to eat potatoes, it is far better to eat them hot than cold in a potato salad and the same goes for white rice (as in sushi) or pasta (as a cold pasta salad).

Also take care when freezing bread. As wheat is baked, the cooking process breaks down the starch, making it more digestible. But when you cool it in the freezer, the starch then becomes resistant. Even if you toast the frozen bread, you will still have a much higher content of resistant starch than if you ate fresh bread. You also need to look out for bread baked on site in a shop as it could be made from frozen dough so, again, the starch may become resistant. It's fine if the dough is made fresh from scratch on the premises and cooked straight away but in some shops it is cooked from frozen dough, so it's best to ask.

By adding in the digestive enzymes mentioned on page 136 you may find over time that it becomes easier to manage these resistant starches because your body is able to break them down more easily and there is less fermentation from them. As you have seen above, resistant starches do convey certain health benefits so it would be good to be able to slowly introduce them back into your diet as your digestive health improves.

Fat

There is still lots of confusion surrounding fats because there are some fats that can help with IBS, while others have an extremely negative effect, not only on IBS but also on your general health. So which fats, exactly, are good for us and which should you avoid, especially if you want to overcome IBS?

Omega 3 and Omega 6 Fats

I would encourage you to focus on including Omega 3 fats – both in your diet and in supplement form. There is a common misconception that high amounts of both Omega 3s and Omega 6s are good for your health and it is true that many women do swear by huge doses of evening primrose oil (rich in Omega 6) to help with PMS. However, studies have shown that if we consume very high levels of Omega 6s we actually diminish the already very small levels of health-boosting Omega 3s that we on average glean from our daily diet.

It is estimated that we are getting up to twenty-five times more Omega 6 fats from our diet than Omega 3 and that for good health it should be nearer a ratio of one to one.[13] Some of the men and women I see in my clinic have been taking combinations such as Omega 3, 6 and 9 in supplement form, because they have heard that we need a good balance of all the Omega fatty acids. This is true, but you have to take into account other sources of these fats in your diet. And in our modern diet we tend to consume many more Omega 6 fats that Omega 3.

If you eat a lot of foods containing vegetable oils, your diet is probably very high in Omega 6 already. (You can now have a simple home finger prick blood test to tell you if you have the correct levels of Omega 3 to Omega 6 in your body – see www.naturalhealthprac-tice.com.) Studies show the more Omega 6 you have in your body in relation to Omega 3, the more inflammation your body will produce, which is not good for IBS (see below).

My advice is to increase your intake of oily fish such as salmon, trout, mackerel, tuna (fresh, not canned, as canning reduces the level of Omega 3), sardines, and also of eggs and flaxseeds, and reduce your intake of Omega 6 by cutting down on polyunsaturated vegetable oils like sunflower and corn oil. Olive oil (an Omega 9 fat) is good to use for cooking and extra virgin olive oil for dressings (also see page 131 about Omega 3 supplements).

Saturated Fats

High saturated fat foods may trigger your IBS symptoms. It is thought these high-fat foods cause your stomach to either empty quicker or slower than it should and this can increase muscle spasms.[14] With IBS you can also have a degree of fat malabsorption where your body struggles to absorb fats. This can result in diarrhoea, because food can pass through your system much too quickly. Your stools may also contain higher levels of fat because it is not being absorbed properly and they will tend to look pale and be very smelly because of this (a simple stool test can show you whether your stools contain too much fat, see page 55).

Consuming high levels of saturated fats, especially those found in meat and dairy products, isn't a good idea for your health generally. For IBS sufferers, saturated fats also make it harder for your body to absorb those good Omega 3 fats efficiently, which in turn leads to an increase of inflammation in your body. And of course inflammation in the gut is just what we need to avoid when calming the symptoms of IBS and getting the digestion back to really good working order.

Inflammation is something we should all seek to avoid, but it is more pertinent still if you have IBS. The more inflammation you have in your body, the worse your IBS symptoms can be, especially in relation to pain and cramping.

The easiest way to reduce the saturated fats in your diet is to eat less meat and dairy. But you needn't become a vegetarian to avoid them.

INFLAMMATION

I have mentioned inflammation quite a lot in relation to IBS but it is not only important to control inflammation for your bowel health but also your general health. Increased inflammation has now been linked to many of our degenerative illnesses including heart disease, cancer, diabetes and Alzheimer's.

You do need some inflammation in your body, but it has to be produced at the appropriate time. If your body thinks it is under attack either from bacteria or because you have been injured, then it needs to react quickly and create heat, pain, redness and soreness, basically inflammation, to stimulate your immune system to start off the healing process, causing cells to multiply and divide, to fight the bacteria, or make your blood clot quicker because you have been cut and are bleeding.

But this inflammatory response should happen only occasionally when your body registers there is a crisis. Problems can arise when there is chronic inflammation happening in your body caused by poor diet, stress, lack of exercise and exposure to toxins.

Persistent inflammation can give you pain such as IBS or arthritis, swollen gums, eczema or more 'silent' problems such as heart disease, cancer, diabetes, Alzheimer's and weight gain, especially around your middle . It can also lead to autoimmune problems, such as rheumatoid arthritis, multiple sclerosis and coeliac disease, where the body turns on itself and the inflammatory response ends up attacking its own cells.

To help keep you in good health you must aim to control inflammation.

Eggs and oily fish do contain some saturated fats but also contain the healthy Omega 3 fats so are a good balance. If you are eating meat or chicken then buy free-range or organic grass-fed, as they are going to contain healthier fats than corn-fed animals because of the balance of fats that metabolizes from the food they eat.

Digestive enzyme supplements can help with fat digestion because they contain lipase which is the fat-digesting enzyme (see page 135). And if you are having a fatty meal just have less of it, to reduce the load on your digestive system.

Trans Fats

These are the worst fats of all and should be avoided at all costs. Trans fats were created by the food industry to extend the shelf life of processed foods such as cakes, biscuits and fast foods. They are produced by chemically altering liquid oils to make them into solids by passing hydrogen through the oil at a high temperature and under pressure. They have no nutritional benefit to you whatsoever, and it's just not worth having them in your diet.

Trans fats act like a plastic, which means our bodies do not know what to do with them, and they can cause all sorts of unhealthy processes to occur. Not only do trans fats create more inflammation in the body but they also block the absorption of the essential fatty acids, which are needed to produce an anti-inflammatory response in your body. They are a double negative when it comes to trying to control inflammation.

A number of countries and cities (Denmark, Switzerland, Austria and New York) have banned trans fats not only in food products but also in restaurants and fast food outlets, but UK officials say a ban would be too difficult to implement, so just be vigilant and read ALL food labels. Trans fats will be listed on food labels as 'hydrogenated' or 'partially hydrogenated vegetable oil'.

Sugar

In my opinion, added sugar in food is the biggest cause of our health problems today and whether you are eliminating digestive problems, aiming to lose weight or get your health back you have to think about eliminating or drastically reducing the amount of added sugar in your diet. Not only can sugar cause weight gain but it also increases the risk of Type 2 diabetes, heart disease and cancer.

Sugar is added (without you realizing) to many foods which means we consume an average of around forty-six teaspoons of it every day.[15] It is added to both savoury and sweet foods and offers zero nutritional benefits, just empty calories.

Sugar is added to savoury foods like tomato ketchup and soups, mayonnaise and salad dressing, and even a supposedly 'healthy' fruit yoghurt can contain as much as eight teaspoons of added sugar. In particular, watch out for 'healthy' looking breakfast cereals – a portion can sometimes contain more sugar than a doughnut! (11.1g or 3 teaspoons in a small bowl of cereal compared to 8.6g in one doughnut.)

It is not only the longer-term effects of sugar that you must consider but, on a daily basis, living on a rollercoaster of sugar highs and lows will give you symptoms such as tiredness, mood swings, anxiety, tension, headaches, difficulty concentrating and feeling more stressed (see Chapter 7). And because this rollercoaster makes your body produce more of the stress hormones, adrenaline and cortisol, in response to low blood sugar (hypoglycaemia), sugar can trigger IBS symptoms, in particular bloating and flatulence.

Tips for Beating Sugar Cravings

- Eliminate sugar and foods and drinks with added sugar. This might seem difficult at first but there are so many other choices of the same products without added sugar. By removing refined sugar from your diet, you can avoid living on a sugar rollercoaster, with your blood sugar soaring up and crashing down during the day. Eat little and often, and go no longer than three hours without eating. This means having breakfast, lunch and dinner as well as a snack mid-morning and one in the afternoon. By eating regularly like this you avoid the blood sugar drops and then your body does not have to create a craving to send you off for a quick fix.

- Have breakfast – this literally means 'breaking the fast' because you have been without food overnight. If you miss breakfast, by about 11am your blood sugar will have dropped so low that you are desperate for that cup of coffee and a pastry. Start the day as you mean to go on, eat within one hour of waking and then keep eating little and often.

- Have protein with every meal. Protein helps to lower the GI of a carbohydrate, reducing the risk of a quick spike in blood sugar and then a crash. Protein can be animal (like fish or eggs) or vegetable (like nuts or quinoa) and this combination will help to make you feel fuller for longer and more satisfied with what you have eaten.

- Get moving – exercise is a brilliant way to reduce sugar cravings.

- Change your patterns. If you always fill up your car at the same garage and then buy chocolate or walk past the same bakery every day and buy a pastry, then you need to change your routine.

- Get a good night's sleep. A good night's sleep is important because lack of sleep disrupts hormones, triggering changes in metabolism and an increase in appetite. Tiredness triggers sugar cravings so take a power nap for no longer than twenty minutes instead of reaching for the biscuit tin.

- Don't eat sweets while watching the TV or working on the computer. Scientists talk about 'mindless or unconscious eating' because you can end up eating a lot without realizing it.

- Enjoy it! If you have a sugar craving then buy the highest-quality version of that product you can, so not cheap chocolate but good organic dark chocolate. Sit down, do nothing else at the same time and savour the texture and taste of that food and enjoy it. Acknowledge that you are eating that food and let go of the guilt.

- Aim for the 80/20 rule. If you eat well 80 per cent of the time then the other 20 per cent at birthdays and holidays, your body will cope. So you could give yourself a 'cheat day' one day a week and eat anything you want. Interestingly, if you give yourself permission to eat sweet foods, you can end up eating less of them. If you perceive that these foods are restricted or limited then you want more. It is human nature that if we think we can't have something we want it more!

- Distract yourself. If only chocolate will do, then it is a craving, not hunger, so go for a walk or phone a friend. Cravings can usually last about ten minutes, so ride it out.

- Have a drink of water or herbal tea. Often drinking something can curb sweet cravings because the liquid makes you feel fuller. You may be reaching for a sugar fix when actually what you really need to do is rehydrate your body.

- Don't shop on an empty stomach. Shopping when you are hungry is a bad idea as it makes you far more likely to binge on calorie-rich, sugary foods. Make a list of exactly what you need and stick to it.

- You can still make homemade cakes and other baked goods and I have included some in the recipes on pages 100–7 and shown you what ingredients you can use.

- As well as the sugar contained in the foods you eat, you need to wean yourself off the sugar you add to hot drinks. You could add a small amount of maple syrup (needs to be the real maple syrup not maple-flavoured syrup) and then gradually reduce the amount until you can drink it completely unsweetened.

THE DIET PLAN

For those who do not wish to create their own exclusion diet I have developed a seven-day Diet Plan to give you a healthy start. I know from experience that, for the majority of IBS sufferers, it works. I would suggest you eat in this way for a two-week period and monitor your symptoms during this time. I have provided daily meal options with recipes but don't feel you have to stick to the meal plan. I will outline the principles of this diet so you can create your own recipes instead, if you wish, or mix and match my recipes with your own.

As wheat and dairy are the most common culprits with not only IBS symptoms but also general digestive problems, as outlined in Chapter 8, I have omitted both of these from the recipes. You may want to take out the other gluten grains such as barley and rye if you have tested positive for gluten sensitivity or suspect this is one of your symptom triggers (and if you are coeliac then you will need to exclude all gluten). I have included oats in the Diet Plan as they do not contain gluten and so are usually good for most people. However, they do contain a protein similar to gluten called avenin, so you can keep an eye out for whether you might be sensitive. (If you are coeliac then choose oats that are labelled 'gluten-free' as some of the regular oats can be slightly contaminated with gluten from wheat, rye or barley during the milling process.)

Dairy foods are omitted from the Diet Plan but don't worry about leaving them out for two weeks because you will get calcium from a multivitamin and mineral (see Chapter 6 on supplements), plus there are many other non-dairy foods that contain calcium in my Diet Plan, such as tinned salmon and sesame seeds (see list on page 71).

If you have looked at IBS diets before you will see that there is no agreement about what to eat (some say high fibre, some say low fibre, for example) and this is also true among the experts and the scientists. So I have used my knowledge and over thirty years of experience in nutrition to devise this Diet Plan to give you the quickest relief from your symptoms in the shortest space of time. We are all different and what may be a difficult food to digest for someone with IBS may be fine for another IBS sufferer. The point of following the Diet Plan is to find out what affects *you* so that you then know what happens when you eat certain things. There may also be times that you can 'get away' with eating a particular food and other times when that same food may cause a problem. This could be because you are tired or stressed. But at least, over time, you will get to know your own body and what it can cope with and when.

The long-term goal is for you to be able to reintroduce most foods because your gut has calmed down and is not 'irritable' any more, and you may find that as long as you don't overdo the amount of certain foods you will cope really well.

I have outlined seven days of breakfasts, lunches and dinners with mid-morning and mid-afternoon snacks. You are to repeat the seven days for another week and keep track of your symptoms in the chart below.

My suggestion is to try this plan first and if your symptoms improve dramatically then wonderful. If not then the next step would be to try the FODMAP diet, outlined later in this chapter. It's quite a bit more restrictive, which is why I always encourage this simple diet first.

THE LOW-DOWN

What the Diet Plan avoids:

Grains. Wheat products – including bran, couscous, semolina, wheatgerm, spelt and durum – and also barley and rye.

Dairy foods, and not just those that contain lactose, like milk. This is because removing dairy foods in IBS seems to help with the symptoms even in those IBS sufferers who are not lactose intolerant. Also avoid sheep's and goat's milk products.

Sweeteners. Sugar, fructose, fruit juice concentrates, sorbitol, xylitol, agave, glucose (although glucose is theoretically OK for IBS, it is in my opinion not good for your general health because of its effect on blood sugar, see page 123) and artificial sweeteners.

Caffeine. Caffeinated drinks like tea, coffee and colas and also decaffeinated coffee, as this still contains stimulants that can irritate your digestive system, even once the caffeine is removed (decaff tea is fine). Alcohol and fizzy drinks need to be avoided too and that includes carbonated (sparkling) water at the moment as this can give you more gas and cause bloating.

Chocolate. This is a problem because it will often contain milk and sugar. Even dark chocolate contains one of the stimulants (theobromine) found in coffee. It's not as strong as in coffee and so some people will be able to gradually add it back in after the two weeks.

Red meat. This is high in saturated fats and is also a difficult food to digest. It is associated with problems such as diverticulitis (see page 195) and bowel cancer so is best avoided.

Gas-producing foods. Beans (like chickpeas, lentils and kidney beans) and certain vegetables such as broccoli, Brussels sprouts, cauliflower, cabbage, onions and leeks.

Fruit. Have just three portions of fruit a day and avoid fruit juice while on the Diet Plan. And eat more citrus fruits, berries, grapes and bananas than apples, pears and dried fruit.

What you should eat on the Diet Plan:

Go organic. When you have digestive problems it is a good idea to eat foods that are as high in nutrients as possible, as you may not be absorbing these quite as well as your body needs you to. Likewise, your gut might not be producing nutrients like the B vitamins, so organic foods can give a helping hand. You will also be reducing your exposure to chemicals such as pesticides and this is important as your body is trying to heal itself and anything you can do to lessen the burden of chemicals is a good thing.

Non-wheat grains. Include rice, buckwheat (not related to wheat although the name implies it), oats, millet, corn and quinoa (quinoa is not actually a grain but a seed and cooks like rice) in your diet. Instead of wheat flour for cooking you can use rice flour, buckwheat flour, almond flour and gram flour (made from chick-peas) or mixtures of these.

You can get rice noodles and also pasta made from corn so there are plenty of choices nowadays – very different from when I started in the field of nutrition many years ago. Buckwheat noodles are also good, although heavier than those made from rice, but be careful to read the labels as the manufacturers will often add wheat to buckwheat noodles.

Get used to reading the ingredients of such foods as condiments. For example, lots of soy sauces contain wheat so it is often better to look for wheat-free tamari soy sauce. I know you can buy gluten-free breads and other baked foods but the ingredients have, in general, appalled me. The aim seems to be to make the food 'gluten-free' and disregard the health aspects of the food, so other ingredients such as sugar, artificial colours and flavours are often added. This is not the right approach when it comes to IBS. You do want to avoid gluten over the next two weeks but still to eat healthily. Again, read labels carefully.

Dairy substitutes. You have many choices here including soya milk and rice milk. Buy organic where possible and especially for soya because if the soya is organic it won't be genetically modified. You can also use almond or cashew nut milk and if you can't buy these they are easy to make (see the almond cream recipe on page 100).

'Good' sweeteners. Include maple syrup (but make sure it is pure maple syrup and not maple-flavoured syrup containing high fructose corn syrup, which is definitely not good for IBS or your general health), barley malt syrup and rice syrup.

Butter substitutes. I always say that butter is healthier than margarine because it is more of a natural product, but you need to remove all dairy on the Diet Plan over the next two weeks. So in this instance, you can use margarine but get a good quality one that does not contain hydrogenated fats. Unfortunately, even the fat in margarine may cause symptoms in IBS, so use it sparingly. You can also use nut butters (peanut or almond butter) or tahini (sesame seed paste) as a spread. I know nut butter and tahini contain fats but they are usually a healthier and less processed fat than that found in margarine. As you are cutting out wheat for these two weeks, you won't need spreads too much.

If you like sweet spreads, there are some lovely pure fruit jams (no added sugar) on the market and you may be able to tolerate the berry ones, such as strawberry. These are not the diabetic jams that are often sweetened with sorbitol, which is not good for IBS.

TOP TEN FOODS FOR IBS

I know you are most often told what not to eat with IBS so I thought it would make a pleasant change to put together a list of those foods that are really helpful to include, and most of these foods are included in my Diet Plan recipes. I have chosen my top ten and these not only help reduce the IBS symptoms but also show what a varied and interesting diet you can have even as you heal your digestion.

1. Oats

Oats contain soluble fibre, the kind of fibre that is more soothing and less harsh on your digestive system (and helps reduce cholesterol). They also provide good amounts of zinc, magnesium, calcium, iron and the B vitamins, B1, B2 and B6. Oats are easy to digest and have a low glycaemic index which means that they hit your bloodstream slowly and help keep your blood sugar steady, which in turn helps with weight control, giving you more sustained energy during your day.

They make the perfect breakfast but are versatile enough to be used in many other ways. You can also grind the oat flakes into a flour and use this as a substitute for wheat flour in cakes, pancakes and flapjacks. I also use ground oats as a topping for crumble. Oats can also be made into oat milk, and can be used as a non-dairy alternative to milk.

I would suggest you don't use instant porridge oats because in order to make them 'instant' they are pre-cooked and dried, so you will not get as much benefit in terms of energy and blood sugar balance because they will be digested quicker. In addition, sweeteners are often added to instant oats, and these should be avoided.

2. Quinoa

Quinoa (pronounced keen-wah) is a seed although it cooks like a grain and is a good source of vegetable protein. You may not have tried it before so I have described how to cook it below because it is always good to have choices and not feel restricted in what you are eating.

Quinoa originates from Peru and Bolivia, where it is still grown today. It contains high levels of minerals, is rich in vitamins and can be used as a change from rice. Quinoa is easy and quick food to prepare. It has a protein content of between 12 and 18 per cent and unusually for the vegetable world has a complete set of essential amino acids. It is high in both magnesium and iron and is easy to digest and gluten-free, with a good amount of fibre.

For thousands of years, quinoa used to be the staple food of the Incas. It is very versatile and can be used in both savoury and sweet dishes. The easiest way to cook it is to bring two cups of water to a boil with one cup of quinoa, covering at a low simmer and cooking for 14–18 minutes. It is served instead of rice, pasta or potatoes and the leftovers could be used for breakfast as a breakfast mix topped with berries.

Quinoa can also be sprouted like alfalfa or mung beans. Sprouting increases the vitamin and mineral content and this means that it can be used raw in salads as you would other sprouts. Alternatively, a mix of different sprouts would make a good addition to any raw dish.

3. Eggs

Eggs are a first class protein meaning that they contain all the essential amino acids. Over the years eggs have gone up and down in popularity but for me they have always been a good food. Eggs contain good amounts of vitamin D and also Omega 3 fatty acids. And contrary to a myth that has lasted for many years they do not raise cholesterol, have no connection with increasing the risk of heart disease and there is no limit to how many you can eat.[16]

As well as a good amount of vitamin D and Omega 3 fatty acids, eggs also contain two carotenoid antioxidants, lutein and zeaxanthin, and research has shown that these two substances are important in the prevention of age-related macular degeneration and cataracts. Eggs also contain good amounts of the B vitamins including folic acid.

Just remember to be careful as to how you prepare your eggs, because often it is the foods that are added in cooking that are the problem rather than eggs – scrambled eggs in restaurants are often made with milk or cream. I would suggest that you substitute milk and cream with water when you make scrambled eggs, which is how I make them anyway, but you could add rice milk if you wanted. The same goes for omelettes: leave out the cheese and fill them with a good quantity of delicious vegetables. My recommendation would be to always choose organic eggs where possible and if not then at least go for free-range as the nutritional value of the eggs will be better than eggs from caged hens (and better for the birds too).

4. Oily fish

Oily fish is important for its Omega 3 fatty acids as well as other dietary benefits. Do include white fish, too, for variety, but remember the oily ones will give you the most benefit. Oily fish include salmon, mackerel, herring, pilchards and tuna (fresh tuna, not canned, because the oils are lost in the canning process).

Oily fish provide us with important Omega 3 oils that have anti-inflammatory properties (see page 130) and are so helpful with IBS. Omega 3 fatty acids can help lower blood pressure, reduce the risk of heart disease, soften the skin, increase immune function, increase metabolic rate, improve energy, help with arthritis because of their anti-inflammatory effect and help with skin problems such as eczema. Oily fish is also a good source of vitamin D, and some types also contain good amounts of selenium, vitamins B3, B6 and B12 and also vitamin D.

The Department of Health recommends that we should double our intake of Omega 3 oils by eating oily fish two to three times a week. But concerns have been raised about mercury intake from oily fish. I can reassure you that research shows that the health benefits from eating oily fish definitely outweigh the risks, and that in fact we are not eating enough fish in general. The Harvard School of Public Health has shown that eating about six ounces of mackerel each week can reduce the risk of death from heart disease by a third.

5. Berries

Berries are good for IBS because they are less likely than other fruits to ferment in the intestines, causing gas and bloating. They are low on the FODMAP diet (see page 108) because they contain less fructose than some fruits, such as apples. Include different berries for variety, like strawberries, blueberries and raspberries. Frozen berries are fine if you can't get fresh ones.

Berries are good for IBS but they are also really beneficial for your general health. These fruits that herald the start of summer in Britain are packed with phytochemicals (plant chemicals) that protect against cancer and heart disease. Berries contain high concentrations of ellagic acid, which has been shown to prevent healthy cells from becoming cancerous, and isothio-cyanates, which can both prevent and kill cancer development in the cervix and oesophagus.

These and other antioxidant compounds in berries, such as quercetin and anthocyanins, also help to cut the risk of cardiovascular disease by reducing the amount of 'bad' LDL cholesterol in the bloodstream and lowering the risk of throm-bosis. Lab tests have also shown them to be anti-inflammatory which is good for your general health and in particular IBS.

6. Almonds

I am mentioning almonds in particular here, but other nuts can be helpful as well, including walnuts and pine nuts.

Almonds are especially helpful for IBS because you can use almond milk as a substitute for dairy while you are experiment-ing with your diet and you can also use ground almonds as a flour in most recipes (like for like with wheat), thus avoiding grains completely in a recipe if need be.

As well as their versatility, almonds have particular health benefits. They are a good source of protein and monounsatu-rated fat and also contain nine essential nutrients including calcium, riboflavin (B2), niacin (B3) and vitamin E.

Almonds can also give you a sense of fullness, reduce hunger and help curb cravings so they're ideal when you are weaning yourself off cakes and biscuits.[17]

7. Tofu

Beans are going to be difficult to eat when you have IBS because they can cause flatulence and bloating but it may be worth you trying to see whether you can tolerate tofu. Tofu is of course made from soya beans but because of the way it is made, it is very easy to digest. It is versatile to use in recipes as it is quite bland and so takes up the flavours of what you are cooking.

Tofu is often described as a perfect food because it is high in good-quality protein, low in saturated fats, cholesterol-free, easy to digest and carries with it a number of health benefits. Research into the health benefits of tofu, like soya in general, has shown that it can reduce the risk of heart disease because it lowers LDL ('bad') cholesterol. Tofu is also rich in phytoestrogens and research has shown that women who eat a diet rich in phytoestrogens have fewer hot flushes and night sweats.

The texture of tofu varies from soft to firm to extra-firm. Soft tofu has a smooth texture and is more suited for salad dressings, sauces and desserts, while firm and extra-firm tofu are best for baking, stir frying and grilling.

8. Rice Milk

I have included rice milk as a good food for IBS because it is easy to digest and a good substitute for dairy milk, either used on its own or in cooking. But you must check the labels on the rice milk as you want a product with as few ingredients as possible. I would always go for the organic versions and avoid any that contain sweeteners (as the rice milk is naturally sweet anyway) and any other additives if you are not clear what they are.

In cooking you can substitute rice milk for dairy milk in the same amounts.

9. Sweet potatoes

This could have been potatoes, but they do not count as one of your five a day fruit and vegetables, so I thought it would be good to include sweet potatoes because these often get forgotten as a vegetable, yet they are really easy to cook and quite delicious. They are also good because they can often satisfy a need for something sweet, especially when baked.

Sweet potatoes belong to the Convolvulaceae or morning glory plant family and are different from yams, with which they are often confused, which are root vegetables belonging to the Dioscoreae family. Sweet potatoes are packed full of nutrients and are an excellent source of beta-carotene, vitamin C, manganese, vitamin B6, potassium and iron. They are also a good source of dietary fibre.

There are about 400 different varieties of sweet potato and the skin and flesh can vary in colour, with white, yellow, orange, deep purple and pink varieties. The most common is the yellow-orange variety, which is slightly longer than an ordinary potato and tapered at the ends. The orange colour is due to the beta-carotene content which gives the sweet potato valuable antioxidant properties. Your body can produce vitamin A from beta-carotene and it is thought that the beta-carotene from sweet potatoes is more easily utilized than that from dark, leafy vegetables.

The purple sweet potato has been found to have the highest antioxidant activity of all the sweet potatoes and in one study the antioxidant activity (anthocyanins coming from the purple colour) was over three times higher than that of blueberries.

Try to buy organic sweet potatoes so that you do not have to peel them because, as with most fruit and vegetables, most of the goodness is in the skin and with sweet potatoes the antioxidant activity is three times higher in the skin than in the flesh.

10. Flaxseeds

Flaxseeds (also known as linseeds) can be very helpful for IBS. They are about the size of sesame seeds and contain good amounts of protein and Omega 3 fatty acids and also lignans, which have antioxidant properties and can have a balancing effect on hormones (both for men and women) because of their phytoestrogen properties.

Flaxseeds are helpful for IBS as they have a very soothing affect on the digestive system. I know I have mentioned them on page 187 as a remedy for constipation when used as whole seeds but if used as ground seeds they can be helpful for IBS in general (constipation or diarrhoea). The fibre in the seeds absorbs water and forms a soothing gel-like substance that can stabilize the passage of foods through the intestines, neither too fast or too slow.

I would suggest you buy organic ground flaxseeds (freshly ground would be better, but I know this can be impractical) that come in vacuum-sealed packs which can be kept in the fridge. Ground flaxseeds can be added to porridge in the morning or added to cakes or breads. You can also try one tablespoon of ground flaxseeds in water in the morning to see if they help soothe your bowel. If you have diarrhoea predominant symptoms then maybe try one teaspoon first to see how your gut reacts.

Now that you are familiar with the principles of the Diet Plan, you can start following the meal plans and recipes on pages 98–107. Before you start, make a note of your symptoms in the table below (or photocopy the table if you would rather not write in the book) and then complete the second table after two weeks.

SYMPTOMS BEFORE STARTING THE DIET PLAN

	None	Severe	Moderate	Mild
Abdominal cramping/ pain or spasms				
Flatulence				
Bloating				
Constipation				
Diarrhoea				
Burping				
Nausea				
Relief on passing stools				
Mucous in stools				
Headaches				
Tiredness				
Frequent toilet visits				

SYMPTOMS AFTER TWO WEEKS ON THE DIET PLAN

	Mild	Moderate	Severe	None
Abdominal cramping/ pain or spasms				
Flatulence				
Bloating				
Constipation				
Diarrhoea				
Burping				
Nausea				
Relief on passing stools				
Mucous in stools				
Headaches				
Tiredness				
Frequent toilet visits				

If there is a considerable difference in symptoms after just two weeks, then you have a choice: you can either enjoy the relief from the IBS symptoms and carry on eating this way for longer or you can gradually reintroduce some foods and see what happens to your symptoms. Try eating just small amounts in the first instance and see how you feel. Remember, it may not only be the type of food that you eat but the quantity of that food, so if you eat a lot of a particular food your body may find it hard to deal with.

The best way to reintroduce foods is to start by adding in spelt, which is an 'ancient wheat' – have small amounts over two days and see how you feel. There is gluten in spelt but it is generally much easier to tolerate than the gluten in wheat. If you do not get a return of symptoms then stick with the spelt and add in another food in small quantities such as organic plain live yoghurt. The yoghurt will contain beneficial bacteria and very little, if any, lactose and in this way you are gradually trying 'gentle' foods first to see what the reaction is. Goat's cheese is often easier for people to digest than cow's cheese, and you can also buy goat's butter and yoghurt. Feta is a sheep's cheese and again might be easier on the digestion as you start to introduce more variety back into your diet.

THE DIET PLAN MENU

Choose from the seven-day meal plan below for two weeks.

	Day 1	Day 2	Day 3
Breakfast	Porridge with frozen berries and ground flaxseeds	Scrambled eggs with grilled tomatoes	Gluten-free muesli with soya milk
Mid-morning snack	Rice cakes with mackerel paté	Banana and sunflower seeds	Oat cakes
Lunch	Quinoa salad with avocado, cucumber, parsley and radish	Vegetable frittata (recipe) and a cherry tomato salad	Jacket potato with tuna, broad beans, mint, dill and olive oil
Mid-afternoon snack	Orange or pear and brazil nuts	Gluten-free sugar-free fruit bar	Bowl of mixed berries with almond cream (recipe)
Dinner	Vegetable and prawn stir fry (recipe)	Grilled mackerel with roasted beetroot and crunchy salad	Rice noodles with tofu and vegetables (recipe)

Day 4	Day 5	Day 6	Day 7
Poached eggs on gluten-free bread	Porridge with ground seeds	Sugar-free corn flakes with soya milk	Puffed rice with berries and almond milk
Gluten-free crackers with peanut butter	Smoothie with berries, half a banana and soya yoghurt	Blueberries and a small handful of cashew nuts	Rice cakes with non-dairy butter, such as nut butter
Butternut squash soup (recipe) and Sun-dried tomato bread (recipe)	Sardines and tomatoes on gluten-free toast	Buckwheat pancakes filled with vegetables (recipe)	Omelette with mushrooms sautéed in olive oil and balsamic vinegar with a green salad
Carob brownies (recipe)	Almond cookies (recipe)	Soya yoghurt with berries	Banana and mixed nuts and seeds
Asian salmon with steamed vegetables (recipe)	Fish cakes (recipe)	Stir fried rice with vegetables	Mediterranean baked fish (recipe) with green beans

THE RECIPES

ALMOND COOKIES
Makes 20–30 small cookies (20 minutes)

110g ground almonds
300g gluten-free flour
125ml softened coconut oil
1 egg
125ml pure maple syrup
1 tsp vanilla extract

1. Preheat oven to 180°C/350°F/Gas 4.
2. Combine all ingredients in a food processor to make a stiff dough.
3. Roll out dough and cut out cookie shapes.
4. Place on baking parchment and bake for 10–12 minutes until golden. Transfer to a wire rack and allow to cool.

ALMOND CREAM
(A few minutes)

Ground almonds
Water
Maple syrup

1. This recipe is really easy – just put ground almonds (this will also work with cashews) into a blender and then gradually add water until you get the texture you want, either thick like a cream or pouring consistency like milk.
2. Add pure maple syrup to taste.

ASIAN SALMON WITH STEAMED VEGETABLES
Serves 4 (20 minutes)

4 small salmon fillets

2 tsp tamari soy sauce (or sea salt if you cannot have tamari)

2 tsp white miso paste (omit if you can't tolerate soja)

1 tsp lime zest

1 garlic clove, crushed

½ tbsp sesame oil

½ tbsp fish sauce (nam pla)

2 cm fresh ginger, grated

4 carrots

4 small heads pak choi

1 pack green beans

1. Preheat oven to 200°C/400°F/Gas 6.
2. Place the fish in an ovenproof dish.
3. In a small bowl, combine the tamari, miso, lime zest, garlic, sesame oil, fish sauce and ginger and pour over the fish.
4. Cover with foil and bake for 8–12 minutes or until just cooked.
5. While the fish is cooking, dice the carrots and chop the vegetables into similar-sized pieces. When the fish is nearly ready, steam the vegetables over boiling water and serve together.

Note: Also delicious with fillets of sea bass, sole or tuna.

BUCKWHEAT PANCAKES FILLED WITH VEGETABLES
Serves 4 (5 minutes)

120g buckwheat flour

2 tsp baking powder

Pinch of salt

1 egg

160ml almond or rice milk

Oil for frying

Vegetables for serving

1. Mix the dry ingredients together.

2. Combine the wet ingredients together and add to the dry mix. Whisk lightly.
3. Lightly oil a pan or griddle and heat until a small drop of water sizzles when dropped.
4. Ladle the batter into the pan and cook for about a minute.
5. Fry on both sides until golden brown.
6. Serve with desired vegetables.

Note: Buckwheat pancakes can be served as a savoury dish with vegetables or you can add chopped cooked spinach and spring onions (plus a little chopped chilli if you are tolerant) to the batter before you cook it. You can have them as a sweet dish, either with just maple syrup and a squeeze of lemon or topped with blueberries and almond cream (see recipe on page 100 for almond cream).

BUTTERNUT SQUASH SOUP
Serves 4 (30 minutes)

Olive oil
1 butternut squash, peeled, deseeded and diced
1 sweet potato, peeled and diced
2 carrots, peeled, trimmed and sliced
Pinch of cinnamon and/or nutmeg
Vegetable stock (organic, gluten-free)
Salt and pepper

1. In a large saucepan, gently fry the vegetables and spices in olive oil for a few minutes.
2. Add enough hot vegetable stock to cover the vegetables and bring to the boil. Then reduce the heat and simmer gently for 10 minutes, or until the vegetables are cooked.

3. Remove from heat and blend half the vegetables with the stock into a desired consistency (if you prefer a smooth soup blend all the veg).
4. Return to the pan, mix together, season and serve.

Note: If you can tolerate coconut then you can use half stock, half coconut milk or add toasted coconut flakes before serving to give it a lovely tropical flavour.

CAROB BROWNIES
Makes 16 (40 minutes)

100g gluten-free flour or almond flour
5 tbsp carob powder
Pinch of salt
Handful of walnuts (optional)
250ml pure maple syrup
125ml vegetable oil (corn oil works well)
2 eggs
1 tsp pure vanilla extract

1. Preheat oven to 180°C/350°F/Gas 4. Grease and line a 20-cm (8-inch) square baking tin.
2. Mix together all the dry ingredients. Mix together the wet ingredients and stir into the dry ingredients until blended well.
3. Place in the baking tin and bake for about 30 minutes, until a knife inserted into the centre comes out clean. Allow to cool before cutting into 16 pieces and eating.

FISH CAKES
Makes 12 (30 minutes)

550g potatoes	1 tbsp capers, chopped
60ml rice milk	1 tsp lemon zest
1 bay leaf	30g chopped parsley
1 garlic clove	Sea salt and pepper
Peppercorns	Flour for dusting (rice or oat)
225g smoked undyed haddock	15ml olive oil

1. Boil the potatoes in lightly salted water for about 20 minutes.
2. In another pot, boil the milk, bay leaf, clove of garlic and some peppercorns. Add the haddock, reduce the heat and simmer for 5 minutes. Flake the fish into a bowl. Reserve the poaching milk.
3. While the potatoes are hot, mash with the poaching milk, add chopped capers, lemon zest and parsley. Season and divide the mixture into about 12 flattened balls.
4. Cover the fishcakes lightly with flour and fry in a lightly oiled hot pan for about 5 minutes on each side.
5. Serve with a rocket salad with an orange and sesame dressing.

GLUTEN-FREE SUN-DRIED TOMATO BREAD
Makes 1 loaf (preparation time 10 minutes, baking time 50–60 minutes)

250g gluten-free flour	1 tsp tomato purée
1 tsp salt	2 tbsp olive oil (use oil from
3 tsp gluten-free baking powder	sun-dried tomatoes)
290ml soya milk with a squeeze	50g sun-dried tomatoes in oil
of lemon juice (to mimic	(6–8), coarsely chopped
buttermilk)	Large handful of mixed seeds
3 eggs	(optional)

1. Heat oven to 180°C/350°F/Gas 4. Grease a 22.5 x 10 cm (9 x 4 inch) loaf tin.
2. Mix flour, salt and baking powder in a large bowl and make a well in the centre.
3. In a jug, thoroughly mix the milk, eggs, tomato purée and oil.
4. Pour wet ingredients into dry and fold together gently. Then add sun-dried tomatoes and most of the seeds and mix.
5. Pour mixture into prepared tin and sprinkle with remaining seeds. Bake for 50–60 minutes, until a skewer inserted into the centre comes out clean. Cool on a wire rack.

Note: If you cannot find a gluten-free flour use 160g rice flour, 40g potato flour, 30g tapioca flour, 20g maize flour and 2 tsp xantham gum. Xanthum gum is an essential component of gluten-free baking, helping to improve the crumbly texture associated with most gluten-free breads.

If you cannot find a gluten-free baking powder, use a mix of equal parts cream of tartar, potassium bicarbonate (or sodium bicarbonate) and either brown rice flour or arrowroot. Keep in a screw-top jar.

MEDITERRANEAN BAKED FISH
Serves 2 (25 minutes)

Handful of sun-dried tomatoes, finely chopped
Handful of black olives, pitted and roughly chopped
Handful of pine nuts
2 tbsp fresh marjoram or basil leaves, chopped
Olive oil
Sea salt and pepper
2 fish fillets (firm white fish, trout or salmon)

1. Preheat oven to 200°C/400°F/Gas 6.

2. Mix together the sun-dried tomatoes, olives, pine nuts and marjoram or basil with a little olive oil and sea salt.
3. Make a 'sandwich' of the fish fillets with the tomato and olive mix as the 'filling'.
4. Season and bake at the top of the oven for about 20 minutes, or until the fish is cooked. Serve with green beans.

RICE NOODLES WITH TOFU AND VEGETABLES
Serves 4 (10 minutes)

> *1 tbsp olive oil*
> *1 tbsp grated fresh ginger*
> *Packet of organic tofu, diced and lightly coated in a mix of crushed fennel and mustard seeds*
> *Pack of rice noodles or pure buckwheat noodles, cooked as per instructions on packet*
> *Grated courgettes*
> *Grated carrots*

1. Heat the oil in a wok or large frying pan and add the ginger. Cook until lightly brown, stirring constantly.
2. Add the tofu and cook until brown. Add the noodles and vegetables and stir fry until the vegetables are soft.

VEGETABLE AND PRAWN STIR FRY
Serves 4 (less than 15 minutes)

> *½ tbs olive oil*
> *Selection of vegetables, chopped*
> *1 tbs grated fresh ginger*
>
> *200g peeled prawns*
> *Tamari soy sauce*

1. Heat the olive oil in a wok (or any deep pan with curved sides).
2. Add any combination of chopped/sliced vegetables (all colours of peppers, courgettes, mangetout, baby sweetcorn, beansprouts, Chinese cabbage or broccoli).
3. Add the ginger, prawns and a splash of tamari sauce. Stir fry until cooked.
4. Serve with rice or wheat-free noodles or just on its own. You might like to drizzle over a little sesame oil and add chopped coriander or serve with a Chinese-style omelette, which is made simply by whisking eggs and pouring onto greaseproof paper on a baking tray. Sprinkle with sesame seeds and grill until cooked. Serve rolled up and then sliced.

VEGETABLE FRITTATA
Serves 2 (15 minutes)

½ tbsp olive oil	*Handful of peas*
Handful of asparagus tips	*4 eggs*
Handful of baby spinach	*Salt and pepper*

1. Heat the olive oil in a sauté pan with a metal handle and preheat the grill.
2. Add the asparagus to the pan and sauté gently for 5 minutes.
3. Add the spinach and peas and cook for 2 minutes.
4. Roughly beat the eggs with salt and pepper, pour over the vegetable mixture and cook for a further 2–3 minutes.
5. Finish cooking the frittata under the hot grill until the top is set (4–5 minutes).
6. Serve with a cherry tomato salad with a dressing made with lemon juice and zest and extra virgin olive oil.

FODMAP DIET

The FODMAP diet was created by researchers in Australia and is used to improve symptoms of gut disorders such as IBS. It involves eating only non or low FODMAP foods (see below). This is the most extreme diet for IBS and I would definitely recommend that you try my Diet Plan or your own exclusion diet, as outlined earlier in this chapter, before you go down this route because it is very restrictive. Also, as IBS is a functional problem (your bowel is not working properly) not a problem like coeliac disease (where the lining of the intestines has flattened because of a reaction to gluten), the aim should always be to find a cause rather than just treat the symptoms, otherwise you could be eating a very restrictive diet for the rest of your life (see Chapters 3 and 4 on tests for more information on tracking down the cause).

The FODMAP diet means restricting the intake of:

F – Fermentable

O – oligo-saccharides (galacto-oligosaccharides and fructans), for example lentils, chickpeas, kidney beans, broccoli, wheat

D – Disaccharides (lactose), for example milk, yoghurt, soft cheeses

M – Monosaccharides (fructose), for example apples, pears, honey, fruit juices

A – and

P – Polyols (sorbitol and mannitol), for example xylitol, stone fruits

Sounds quite a mouthful, I know, but I will explain what it all means in terms of your food choices. The aim is to take the resistant starch concept (see page 72) one stage further and remove anything from the diet that is highly fermentable in the intestines. This reduces the amount of bloating and flatulence and can also decrease cramping and diarrhoea.

Research has shown that the FODMAP diet has a 20 per cent better effect on IBS symptoms than the standard NICE IBS dietary advice given out.[18] In one study, 82 per cent of the patients following the FODMAP diet had improvements in bloating compared to 49 per cent following the standard advice, 85 per cent improvement in abdominal pain compared to 61 per cent, and 87 per cent improvement in flatulence compared to 50 per cent on the standard dietary recommendations. It has now been suggested that all patients with IBS and even those with inflammatory bowel disease (IBD) should follow this diet.[19]

The aim of this diet is to reduce all the high FODMAP foods and replace them with lower FODMAP ones. I have included a simple table overleaf to show the high and low FODMAP sources.

There are a number of lists of FODMAP foods online and they don't always match, so it is not easy to come up with a definitive list. For you, it may be, for example, that only fructose is an issue and so you would only need to take out the high FODMAP fruits, honey and any foods in which fructose is added as a sweetener. In America, food and drinks can be sweetened with high-fructose corn syrup – in the UK this sweetener would be labelled as glucose-fructose syrup.

One thing to consider is that it may be the *quantity* of a particular food that determines whether it will trigger your symptoms. For example, you may be OK with a small amount of dried fruit (ten raisins, for example) but more than this becomes a problem. So you will need to experiment with your food a bit to see what you are sensitive to, the food and/or the quantity.

If you try the FODMAP diet then do this over a period of six weeks and keep a note of your symptoms. Then gradually introduce one group of foods at a time. So, for example, you could add in the high FODMAP fruits gradually over two to three days and see how you feel. And then do the same for another group of high FODMAP foods.

HIGH AND LOW FODMAP FOODS

	Fruits	Vegetables	Dairy and Dairy Substitutes	Sweeteners	Grains, Beans and Nuts
High FODMAP foods	Apples Apricots Cherries Papaya Peaches Pears Mango Watermelon Fruit juices Dried fruit Tinned fruit High-fructose corn syrup	Avocado Asparagus Beetroot Broccoli Brussels sprouts Cabbage Cauliflower Onions Leeks Mushrooms Peas	Milk from cows, sheep and goats Soft cheeses Yoghurt	Agave Fructose Fruit juice concentrates Honey Isomalt Maltitol Mannitol Sorbitol Xylitol	All beans Pistachios Rye Wheat
Lower FODMAP foods	Bananas Berries Cantaloupe melons Citrus fruits Grapefruit Grapes Honeydew melons Kiwi	Aubergine Carrots Celery Cucumbers Green beans Lettuce Parsnips Potato Pumpkin Squash Sweetcorn Tomato	Brie Butter Camembert Coconut milk Hard cheeses Lactose-free dairy products Rice milk Soya milk Tofu	Barley malt syrup Brown rice syrup Maple syrup	Buckwheat Corn Oats Nuts other than pistachios Quinoa Rice Seeds

The aim is not to be on a low FODMAP diet for life but to use it to ease your symptoms and discover your problem foods. You should be able to gradually reintroduce the foods to your diet and your body should be able to cope with them, especially when you put into place the other recommendations in this book. And you may find that, over time, you only get a reaction to something if you have too much in too short a time.

SUGARS AND SWEETENERS

In theory, sucrose (table sugar) would be OK on the FODMAP diet but I can't recommend you use it or have foods to which it is added as a sweetener, as in my opinion it is one of the worst foods we can have for our general health and can lead to weight gain, diabetes, liver problems, heart disease and cancer (see page 79). Also, artificial sweeteners that don't end in the letters 'ol' are theoretically OK on the FODMAP diet but again I have serious concerns, even more serious than sugar, about using artificial sweeteners. First of all, ironically, they can make you gain weight and increase your appetite, especially when most people are using them thinking they can help control their weight.[20] To explain: because they taste sweet but contain no calories, your body gets confused. When your tongue tastes something sweet your body expects to receive a bulk of calories as a result, but the artificial sweeteners don't provide them! As a result, your body makes you crave those calories from other foods to make up the difference, which means you can end up eating more.

Artificial sweeteners can have an effect on your moods, memory and behaviour.[21] It is thought that artificial sweeteners reduce the antioxidant activity in the brain that protects cells and DNA from damage. They can also have a negative effect on your liver in the long term.

My experience from working in the clinic is that, over time, by limiting sugar and artificial sweeteners, your taste buds will change. You will begin to appreciate the natural sweetness in different fruits and vegetables. Many patients who've reduced their intake of sugar and sweeteners have said that if they have a dessert after not having sugar or artificial sweeteners for a while, they find the dessert far too sweet and don't like the taste. If you do find that you need a sweetener for some foods, try small amounts of maple syrup, brown rice syrup or barley malt syrup as these are healthier alternatives.

DRINKS

We have covered what you should eat to help control the symptoms of IBS but what about what is best to drink?

FRUIT JUICES AND SMOOTHIES

I recommend avoiding all fruit juices, even if they are made from a fruit in the low FODMAP section. Fruit juice is made by removing the juice from the fruit and discarding the fibre, so the effect on your body – especially on your blood sugar – is going to be more immediate and stronger because there is nothing to slow down the effect of the juice. A smoothie should be OK as long as it is made with the fruits that are listed in the low FODMAP section (see page 110), as it is made from the whole fruit and so retains the fibre content.

COFFEE

Coffee stimulates the wave-like muscle contractions – or peristalsis – that move your food through your digestive tract. When you have IBS you do not want to drink something that can increase these contractions.[22] Coffee contains three stimulants that can contribute to problems, one of which is caffeine, the other two being theobromine and theophylline. (This explains why decaffeinated coffee can still stimulate your bowels but to a lesser extent.)

Often people will use coffee as a laxative because it can loosen bowel motions. But if you suffer from diarrhoea, it will worsen the situation. Coffee is also acidic and so can irritate your digestive tract.

The general recommendations for IBS are that you should think about avoiding coffee (caffeinated and decaffeinated) completely.[23] My advice is to eliminate caffeine gradually. Don't suddenly stop overnight as you will suffer withdrawal symptoms, such as headaches, shaking and muscle cramps. It's much better to cut down slowly over a few weeks. Begin by substituting decaffeinated coffee for half of your total intake per day, and gradually switch to all decaffeinated. Then, slowly substitute other drinks, such as herbal teas, until you've removed decaffeinated coffee from your diet, too.

TEA

Tea also contains caffeine but about half the amount found in filtered coffee. Unlike coffee, once the caffeine is removed from tea there are no stimulants left, although it does contain tannin, which can prevent important minerals including iron from being absorbed, so if you are having a cup of tea don't drink it with your meals, and leave half an hour before or after food to have a cup. Green and white teas also contain caffeine (the same amount) but only about a quarter of the amount found in black tea and you may find that you can tolerate a small amount of these. If you go overboard your body will tell you. You could always try decaffeinated green tea as green tea does have beneficial health effects such as good levels of antioxidants and anti-inflammatory effects.

COLAS AND SOFT DRINKS

The trouble with colas and soft drinks is that they usually contain either added sugar or artificial sweeteners and/or caffeine. They are also carbonated so can make you feel even more bloated and gassy. I recommend avoiding these completely.

ALCOHOL

Alcohol can irritate your digestive tract and trigger your IBS. Again, symptoms may differ depending on the alcohol you drink. Some people find beer particularly difficult and others find they can tolerate a small amount of vodka. Dry wines may suit you better than sweet wines and the amount you drink will often come into play too.

GOOD ALTERNATIVE DRINKS

- Herbal teas – peppermint, chamomile and fennel are especially helpful for IBS
- Red bush tea (rooibos) – a tea grown in South Africa which is naturally free from caffeine
- Soya, rice or coconut milks
- Water – drink hot or cold; nice served with a squeeze of lemon or lime juice (if citrus fruits don't trouble your system)

WATER

Drinking plenty of water is important for your digestive system, but I want to be clear that this does not mean you have to drink eight glasses of cold water a day. Your liquid intake can include herbal teas and the fluids that you get with more watery foods such as soups; they all count.

Water is absolutely essential for every function of the body, not just your digestive system. We might be able to survive without food for five weeks but we can't live more than five days without water. We're all made up of more than 70 per cent water and we need every drop to help transport nutrients and waste products in and out of the cells, carry waste out of the body and maintain body temperature.

Water can also have a direct impact on your energy levels – you may be reaching for a sugar fix when what you really need to do is rehydrate your body. And if you want to lose weight, water is essential, since burning fat increases the toxins in your system, which then need to be flushed out by your liver and kidneys. If there isn't adequate water to do this, your body will burn fat less efficiently as this natural function won't be triggered.

But do you know exactly what is in the water that you drink? It is estimated that as many as 60,000 different chemicals now contaminate our water supply. In addition to man-made oestrogens (like xenoestrogens and oestrogens from the contraceptive pill and HRT), a 2004 Environment Agency report found traces of Prozac and seven other drugs in the UK water supply. The standard purification techniques used by most water companies remove the bugs from the water but do not remove all the dissolved chemicals. In attempts to clean the water, other chemicals are often added, including chlorine and aluminium. Not only may these chemicals be toxic in their own right, but chlorine may react with organic waste to form compounds which can increase the risk of cancer of the colon, rectum and bladder.

I am often asked what is the best type of water to drink: tap, bottled or filtered? Also, does it matter what type of container you use to carry the water around in during the day?

Let's start with **tap water**. It is not ideal, in my view, but if you filter it, that helps considerably. Filtered tap water is the cheapest and easiest way to ensure the water you are drinking is relatively clean.

Water filter jugs and bottles are readily available and I would recommend using the filtered water for cooking as well as for hot and cold drinks. Filters can become breeding grounds for bacteria so replace the filter every month and clean the jug at least once a week. A good-quality filter should eliminate or greatly reduce the levels of chlorine and heavy metals such as lead and cadmium, and remove any adverse tastes, colours and smells in the water.

If you want to go to the next level you can buy plumbed-in filters for use in your kitchen sink or you can go for a system which is fitted to your mains water system at home so all your water, including what you are soaking in in the bath, has also been filtered.

When it comes to **bottled water**, you may be surprised to know that not all bottled waters are the same – you need to read the label to see whether it says 'mineral', 'spring' or maybe just 'pure' water:

- **Mineral water** is bottled in its natural underground state and is untreated. It has to come from an officially registered source, conforms to purity standards and carries details of its source and mineral analysis on the bottle.
- **Spring water** is normally taken from one or more underground sources and has undergone a range of treatments, such as filtration and blending.
- **Naturally sparkling water** is water from its underground source with enough natural carbon dioxide naturally occurring to make it bubbly.
- **Sparkling (carbonated) water** will have had carbon dioxide added during the bottling process just as ordinary fizzy drinks do.
- Some **still waters**, if they don't say mineral or spring, and instead say 'pure', 'table' or 'still' on the label, can just be filtered tap water!

- Watch out for **flavoured spring waters**, because although they sound wonderfully natural they can often contain sugar or artificial sweeteners.

So my advice is to choose mineral water when you can when buying bottled water, and to use a filter at home.

I do have concerns about the containers water is generally stored in. We mainly drink water from plastic bottles and a growing number of scientists are concerned about the safety of these products, as chemicals from the plastic can seep into the water. These chemicals are defined as substances that can 'interfere with the synthesis, secretion, transport, binding, action, or elimination of natural hormones in the body that are responsible for development, behaviour, fertility, and maintenance of homeostasis (normal cell metabolism)' and so are not good for your health in general.[24] The most common chemical used to make plastic bottles is BPA (Bisphenol A) and I recommend you reduce your exposure to this by doing the following:

- Use glass bottles instead of plastic where possible
- If you use a plastic bottle choose one that states it is BPA-free
- Don't refill old ordinary plastic bottles, as the risk of BPA leeching into the water will increase the older the bottle and the more damaged it gets
- Don't leave plastic water bottles sitting in direct sunlight as heat increases the leeching effect of the chemicals
- Don't rinse out plastic bottles or containers in very hot water as BPA leeches out fifty-five times faster than normal

'NASTIES' IN YOUR FOOD AND DRINKS

I have covered artificial sweeteners on pages 111–12, and in my opinion you should avoid them completely. But there could be other 'nasties' in your diet that *are* having a negative affect on your IBS symptoms. These can include additives such as preservatives, flavour enhancers, emulsifiers, stabilizers and colourings. Some of these can be natural, but many of them are not and your aim is to help your body heal by reducing the amount of substances it has to deal with and spend time and energy eliminating.

As a rule, if a food or drink has a long list of chemical-sounding names or E numbers then I would avoid it as it can be a long way from being natural. (E numbers are used within Europe as codes for the different additives that are allowed in foods and drinks.) Basically, you need to become a food-label detective!

Some of the E numbers are from a natural source such as E160B annatto, which is derived from the seeds of the achiote tree and is used as a yellow-orange food colour, whereas E102 is tartrazine, an artificial yellow colour that has been associated with allergic reactions and possibly hyperactivity in children. Nowadays most manufacturers will list natural food additives with their name rather than the E number because E numbers generally elicit negative associations and it can be a good selling point to have natural additives rather than artificial ones.

But there is a group of additives which need special mention for IBS and these are called excitotoxins. These excitotoxins are defined as toxic molecules that can stimulate nerve cells so that they are damaged or killed. This excessive stimulation causes the release of certain enzymes and over time these enzymes can damage the structure of cells, including the membrane and DNA.

Two well-known substances that act as excitotoxins that you can find in everyday foods and drinks are **MSG** (monosodium glutamate) and **aspartame**. You have glutamate receptors everywhere in your body, including your digestive system, and glutamate is the most abundant neurotransmitter in your brain, whereas aspartate is a neurotransmitter found largely in the spinal cord. Glutamic acid (the source of glutamate) and aspartic acid (the source of aspartate) are classed as non-essential amino acids, meaning that we do not need to get them from our diet because our bodies produce them internally.

These two amino acids can be contained naturally in our foods such as fish and legumes, and because they are bound together with other amino acids they get released at very low levels in the body. The problems start if we consume these substances when they have been added to foods in the forms of glutamate and aspartame, meaning they can get absorbed quickly and at high levels. This can then cause overstimulation of nerve cells.

When digested, aspartame releases methanol and two amino acids, aspartic acid and phenylalanine, into the body. Methanol converts to formaldehyde (a toxin, classed in the same groups of drugs as cyanide and arsenic) and then to formate or formic acid. Amino acids are fundamental constituents of all proteins, and they interact with each other. Amino acids are normally ingested in small quantities in proteins, and in combination with other amino acids. In this case, however, aspartic acid and phenylalanine are being ingested on their own, and in much larger quantities. The result is that they can unbalance the metabolism of amino acids in the brain.

Glutamate is most often found in the form of MSG and is linked with symptoms such as headaches, indigestion, irregular heart rhythms, tingling sensations and IBS. It is used as a flavour enhancer and is often found in Japanese and Chinese food. The effect of MSG has been dubbed 'Chinese Restaurant Syndrome' because of the symptoms people can experience after eating a Chinese meal, including numbness, tingling, facial pressure, headaches and palpitations.

Glutamate is absorbed very quickly in the digestive tract and the excitotoxin affect of the glutamate can cause the intestinal cells to open up, causing leaky gut, leading to problems with immune function and sensitivities to foods (see page 50). Added to this, a magnesium deficiency, which is very common amongst the patients I see in my clinics, can actually cause an increased sensitivity to glutamate.

Removing both MSG and aspartame from the diet for only four weeks in patients who had IBS (and fibromyalgia) resulted in 84 per cent of the patients saying that over 30 per cent of their symptoms had been resolved and it does seem logical that if both glutamate and aspartame are over-stimulating nerve cells then eliminating them from your diet is going to help a condition where pain or hypersensitivity to pain is a predominant symptom.[25]

My advice is to eliminate all MSG from your diet. You will need to read labels carefully – it may not be labelled plainly as MSG. It could instead be listed as the E number E621, or it could be disguised as hydrolysed protein, hydrolysed vegetable protein, vegetable protein or yeast extract. Avoid any label that lists an ingredient as 'hydrolysed', as the process of hydrolysis which breaks down protein into amino acids ends up with the formation of both glutamic and aspartic acid.

Note that glutamate or glutamic acid is not the same as glutamine, which is mentioned on page 134 and is particularly helpful for the digestive tract.

HOW YOU EAT

We all know the phrase 'you are what you eat' so well now, and it's definitely true that your diet is so important to your health. I've provided advice on changes to the food and drink in your diet to help you on your way to better heath, but *how* we eat can often be a crucial factor too, especially when looking to calm the symptoms of IBS. Here are my tips for good eating practice.

CHEW WELL

The digestive enzyme amylase, which is present in your saliva, helps to break down carbohydrates so if these are broken down more efficiently in your mouth when you chew your food, you are going to get less fermentation lower down in your digestive tract. It's important, therefore, that you chew your foods well.

The advice our parents gave us was very good when it comes to digestion – don't speak with your mouth full and chew properly. Some recommendations go as far as saying that we should chew our food until it becomes liquid but I think most of us would give up eating at that rate. But do chew your food well and don't swallow large chunks of food or stuff food in quickly. One patient described her eating pattern as 'inhaling' her food, which is definitely much too quick.

As well as improved digestion, you will get to enjoy your food more if you chew it well, as you will end up improving your taste buds. Also, if you want to lose weight or think you are eating too much, chewing well is really helpful because it takes your brain twenty minutes to register that you are full and if you take your time and eat slowly you will end up feeling satisfied from eating less.

Embrace the concept of 'mindful eating', that is, take your time when you eat and savour the flavours and textures of your food. Try to avoid unconscious eating, when you are concentrating on something else rather than the food. A good example of this is eating in the cinema, where you can get through quite a lot of food and drink and not even really be aware of it, as you mechanically pop food into your mouth while you stare at the screen.

Also, try not to gulp mouthfuls of air and avoid speaking when you have food in your mouth, as that can cause belching. Lastly, don't drink with food. You do not want to dilute those important enzymes in your saliva, so allow thirty minutes before or after a meal before you drink.

DON'T CHEW GUM

Chewing signals to the rest of your digestive system that food is about to be swallowed. It activates your stomach to produce hydrochloric acid ready to break down protein. However, when you chew gum, nothing *is* going to be swallowed so your digestive system gears itself up with no actual food to deal with. It is not good to have hydrochloric acid secreted in your stomach when there is no food present so I strongly advise that you give up the chewing gum.

EAT LITTLE AND OFTEN

When you eat can have a huge impact on your digestive function. You should eat little and often, and not leave longer than three hours without eating. This keeps your blood sugar (glucose) steady and stops it going through highs and lows.

As you eat, your blood sugar (glucose) rises in response to the food. The higher and quicker it rises, the more insulin has to be produced by your pancreas. The higher your blood sugar goes up, the lower it crashes down afterwards. At the drop (and the drop will also occur if you leave longer than three hours between eating) your body will send you off for a quick fix, like a bar of chocolate or a cup of tea and a biscuit, because it needs to lift the blood sugar up again.

This rollercoaster of highs and lows is not good for your general health because we know that high levels of insulin increase the risk of cancer of the bowel, liver, pancreas, ovary and womb.[26] It's also linked to increased risk of breast cancer in women.[27] And if over time you become insulin resistant, where more and more insulin is being produced by the pancreas but the insulin receptors on your cells do not respond effectively to it, then this can increase your risk of diabetes and high blood pressure.

This rollercoaster is particularly bad for your digestive system and can increase IBS symptoms because as your blood sugar drops, your body releases the stress hormones adrenaline and cortisol from your adrenal glands to release your own sugar stores to try to correct the low level of blood sugar (also known as hypoglycaemia). Immediately the stress hormones are released, no matter the cause, energy is diverted away from non-essential areas, for example your digestive system, and pushed towards your arms and legs in order for you to have the energy to run or fight for your life, because adrenaline and cortisol are your fight-or-flight survival hormones.

Energy which should be helping you digest your food efficiently has been moved elsewhere, meaning your food is left sitting there to ferment, causing constipation, bloating and flatulence or it can go the opposite way and you get an attack of diarrhoea (when under stress it is common for people to get loose stools as the rectum relaxes in response to the stress hormones).

So changing *what* you eat to control the symptoms of IBS is important but it is just as important that you time your food intake well. The aim is to have breakfast, lunch and dinner and to have a mid-morning and a mid-afternoon snack to keep those blood sugar levels steady.

Hopefully after reading this chapter you will be thinking about food more positively again. By identifying certain foods and drinks that are contributing to your IBS symptoms you can begin to take control again and not let the IBS control you. It may seem tough and dispiriting to give up certain foods and drinks you enjoy, but the relief you can experience by removing these offending substances will be well worth it. I hope you have also discovered just how many delicious healing alternative foods there are out there – a restricted diet needn't be repetitive and uninspiring.

CHAPTER 6

HOW TO USE SUPPLEMENTS, HERBS AND NATURAL REMEDIES

I have been working in nutrition now for over thirty years and this used to mean just giving dietary recommendations to my patients. But experience has taught me over those years that many people have deficiencies of key nutrients. Even when we try to eat well, we may still be lacking in certain vitamins and minerals because mass-produced food does not always contain the nutrients it did in the past. Compared to the 1930s our fruits and vegetables are depleted in minerals by an average of 20 per cent – magnesium by 24 per cent, calcium by 46 per cent, iron by 27 per cent and zinc by 59 per cent. Meat and dairy products have also become depleted – iron in meat by 47 per cent, iron in milk by over 60 per cent, calcium in cheese in general by 15 per cent and Parmesan cheese by 70 per cent.[1] With IBS there is also the added risk that you may not be digesting food well enough to really get all the key nutrients and minerals from it.

Of course, your diet is the foundation of health and it is important that this is good but supplementing certain key nutrients that we know are helpful for IBS can be useful. You can also make sure that if you are on a dairy-free diet, for example, that your nutrient needs, such as calcium, are taken care of.

We know that up to 50 per cent of people with IBS are not happy with their medical treatment and end up turning to complementary medicine for answers on how to manage their symptoms.[2] So it is important to know then what works and what doesn't so that you don't waste time and money on untested remedies. There is now lots of medical evidence to show which supplements really can make a difference, and I will outline them for you here. I will also show you what to look for when buying supplements.

YOUR SUPPLEMENT PROGRAMME

I would always suggest that you take a multivitamin and mineral as the foundation of your supplement programme. When you eat you are taking in many different vitamins and minerals in combinations and we want to try to mimic this with a food supplement. Many nutrients are dependent on other nutrients for absorption, for example calcium needs vitamin D for efficient absorption, so we want to include these co-factors (as they are called) together in a good multivitamin and mineral supplement. The multivitamin and mineral you take should depend on your age and whether you are aiming to get pregnant or not. So, for women, if you want to get pregnant then your multi should be aimed at helping with fertility but if you are over the age of forty-five then a multi helping to maintain your health in the lead up and through the menopause would be more helpful.

I would suggest that a good everyday supplement programme contains:

- Multivitamin and mineral, containing a range of nutrients including:

  Calcium – 100mg of calcium citrate

  B vitamins – 25mg of each of the B vitamins

  Vitamin D – 300ius of vitamin D as D3

  Vitamin E – 100ius

  Magnesium – 100mg as magnesium citrate

  Zinc – 15mg of zinc

  Selenium – 100mg

  Chromium – 100mg

  Manganese – 5mg
- Vitamin C
- Omega 3 fish oils

I will explain why many of the nutrients contained in the above programme are going to help with your general health as well as IBS. You should then add supplements that are beneficial for IBS and also focus some specific ones depending on whether your IBS symptoms are more shifted towards constipation or diarrhoea. Just as there are many triggers for IBS symptoms, there are many supplements to choose from and it is important to listen to your body and find those which work best for you.

CALCIUM

Calcium is important especially if you have been following a dairy-free diet and although many non-dairy foods contain calcium (see page 71) it is useful to have some extra calcium from your multi.

B VITAMINS

Your multi should also contain the B vitamins, including vitamin B6. B vitamins are good for general health and vitality, and specifically are beneficial for the immune and nervous system, for cell growth, metabolism, stress (a major trigger with IBS, see page 152) and even your skin and hair. Low levels of vitamn B6 have been associated with IBS.[3]

MAGNESIUM

This relaxes the muscles in the bowel and helps prevent cramping and spasm and should be included in good amounts in your multi. You need magnesium for your general health including bone health, blood pressure, immune function and blood sugar balance. It is particularly helpful for IBS if your main symptom is constipation rather than diarrhoea. By relaxing the muscles in your digestive system it helps to move the stool along the bowel smoothly and also helps to soften the stool by increasing the amount of water in your bowel.

One study showed that constipation was not associated with a low intake of fibre or a low intake of water from fluids but was connected to magnesium deficiency and not having enough watery drinks and foods.[4] It is interesting that watery foods that we eat such as vegetables contain good levels of soluble fibre, which we know is helpful for IBS compared to less watery foods such as bread, which contains more insoluble fibre.

VITAMIN D

Vitamin D is important for IBS because it has a balancing effect on your immune function. It is thought that the immune response in the gut with IBS is too strong and is over-reacting to foods, causing pain and cramping.

These days many people are deficient in vitamin D without realizing it. We have alarmingly low levels of vitamin D in the UK; more than 50 per cent of adults have insufficient vitamin D levels.[5] Australians have a one in four deficiency.[6] Those most at risk in the UK are those who do not go out much in the daytime, those who do not expose their skin to the sunlight and women who constantly wear make-up or cosmetics with in-built sun protection. The tone of our skin affects vitamin D production, so the darker our skin, the less vitamin D production, and covering up large areas of skin for religious reasons will also reduce vitamin D production. It is estimated that we need about thirty minutes of exposure to the sun daily to produce a healthy amount of vitamin D.

Natural food sources of vitamin D are few and far between. It is found in oily fish and eggs. A 100g portion of grilled salmon contains 284ius of vitamin D, a 100g portion of tinned pilchards contains 560ius and the yolk of one egg contains about 20ius. Other sources include fortified foods such as margarines and breakfast cereals. In a day we need to get about 600ius from our diet.

There is some concern that most people today are not getting much vitamin D from their diet, especially those who are eating junk food and eating no or very little oily fish or eggs. Scientists are noting a rise in rickets disease in children who are not eating enough vitamin D-rich foods and spending little time outdoors. This is worrying because having good levels of vitamin D is so important for general health as well as IBS.

You have vitamin D receptors in your gut and it has been shown that if someone has a deficient vitamin D level it can increase the risk of developing inflammatory bowel disease.[7] Obviously IBS is not the same as inflammatory bowel disease but research shows that there is mini-inflammation going on in IBS and as vitamin D has an anti-inflammatory effect, this vitamin can be very helpful.

As many people are vitamin D deficient, I think it is one of those nutrients which is important to test for. (You can get a simple home finger prick test for vitamin D. See www.naturalhealthpractice.com) If you are deficient, you should take extra vitamin D on top of your multi for three months and then re-test to make sure that the level is back to normal. Then continue with the multi, which will help to maintain that level of vitamin D.

VITAMIN C

This is a powerful antioxidant that is very helpful for your immune function. In large amounts it can cause diarrhoea so can actually be helpful if you have constipation by gradually increasing your intake. Start with 500mg once a day and gradually increase the amount by 500mg each day until the stools are the consistency that is comfortable. If you suffer predominantly from diarrhoea rather than constipation, then try just 500mg a day and if it doesn't make the diarrhoea worse then try another 500mg the next day. The optimum amount per day for your general health is 500mg twice a day.

You may find that you react differently to different types of vitamin C. The most common form available is vitamin C as ascorbic acid, which is, as the name implies, acidic, and can cause diarrhoea and flatulence. The other form of vitamin C, the kind I use in the clinic, is alkaline and is in the form of an ascorbate. This is much gentler on your body and your digestive system, and allows you to get the health benefits of the vitamin C without creating an acidic environment. (The vitamin C I use in the clinic is NHP's Vitamin C Support.)

OMEGA 3 FISH OIL

We now know that Omega 3 fish oils are important for many aspects of your health including prevention of heart disease, diabetes, obesity, high blood pressure, high cholesterol, neuropsychiatric disorders and eye problems.[8] They are so important because they help to control inflammation in the body and it is now thought that inflammation is the root cause of many of our degenerative health problems in today's world (see page 77).

It is usually thought there is no inflammation connected with IBS but researchers have found a kind of 'mini-inflammation' in the lining of the bowel which can then make your bowel more sensitive and increase pain and cramping.[9] By using certain nutrients that have an anti-inflammatory effect it is possible to help reduce this sensitivity.

Omega 3 fats are found in oily fish (such as mackerel, salmon, and sardines), flaxseeds (linseeds) and soya. Obviously if you are vegetarian you have to rely on flaxseeds or soya for your sources, and unfortunately the levels are lower than they would be in fish. You should also be aware that you'll get even less goodness from these foods if you are stressed, drinking too much alcohol or not getting enough other key nutrients (particularly zinc, magnesium and vitamin B6).

In supplement form you want 770 EPA and 510mg DHA per day of fish oil. If you don't want to take fish oil then take 1,000mg flaxseed (linseed) oil per day. The Omega 3 fish oil I use in the clinic also contains peppermint oil (it is called Omega 3 Support and available from health food shops or www.naturalhealthpractice.com). Peppermint oil has been shown to be extremely beneficial for helping with IBS as it helps to alleviate many of the symptoms including spasms, bloating, trapped wind, constipation and diarrhoea.[10]

OTHER NUTRIENTS AND HERBS FOR IBS

In addition to the supplements above, which I recommend to any patient with IBS for their essential programme, there are a number of other nutrients and herbs that can help control inflammation and so are particularly helpful for IBS. It can end up looking like a long list, so I would see which look like they may be of help to your specific symptoms and try one at a time to see if it has a positive effect for you.

PROBIOTICS

Probiotics are the hot topic of the digestive-health world and it is important to know first if they are helpful and then which ones you should take because there are many to choose from and in different forms (drinks, powders and capsules).

Having an imbalance of good and bad bacteria is very common with IBS: 'Research has provided increasing support for the idea that disturbances of intestinal microflora occur in patients with IBS and may contribute to disease development and clinical symptoms.'[11] Probiotics are the beneficial bacteria that live in your digestive system and there should be a balance of these 'friendly' bacteria which help to control negative bacteria, parasites and yeasts. But these beneficial bacteria can be reduced or eliminated completely by the use of antibiotics, steroids, the contraceptive pill and HRT. Stress, too much sugar and alcohol can also upset the balance.

The delicate balance of these beneficial bacteria is critical for your health because 70 per cent of your immune system is in your gut and your gut is the largest barrier between you and the outside world. Your gut flora weigh around 1kg (2lb) and you have more cells in your gut than you have in the whole of your body, so you can see how important it is to have the correct balance of these beneficial bacteria.

Scientists think that probiotics help with IBS because the disorder could be caused by an imbalance in bacteria within the gut, the effects of having a gastrointestinal infection, having a small intestinal bacterial overgrowth (see page 54) or an overactive immune function in the gut, and probiotics have been proven to help in all these cases.[12]

Your bowel can be so sensitive that it responds to food by releasing inflammatory substances called prostaglandins in the rectum, which can trigger pain and diarrhoea. It is thought that probiotics help reduce this pain because of their anti-inflammatory effect on the body (prebiotics also have this benefit – see below), and in this way they can calm your bowel down and be helpful in controlling the symptoms of IBS.[13] The two most important bacteria for helping to reduce abdominal pain are Lactobacillus acidophilus and Bifidobacteria bifidum.[14]

I would always suggest that for IBS you take probiotics as a supplement rather than a probiotic drink. Many of the drinks available are loaded with added sugar, which is not good for controlling yeasts and other negative bacteria in your gut and is not good for your general health. You want to choose a probiotic that contains both lactobacillus and bifidobacterium strains (about 22 billion in total).

The probiotic I use in the clinic is NHP's Advanced Probiotic Support, which is freeze dried so does not need to be refrigerated and therefore is good when travelling. It contains both lactobacillus and bifidobacterium strains as well as a prebiotic (see below), glutamine (see page 134) and gamma oryzanol (see page 134). It's available from health food shops or www.naturalhealthpractice.com.

PREBIOTICS

Prebiotics are the food that the good bacteria use to thrive on so are useful in helping to make sure that the levels of the beneficial bacteria stay high. They can often help with either constipation or diarrhoea.

Prebiotics boost the levels of the good bacteria bifidobacteria and also lactobacilli and reduce the negative ones such as clostridia (for example C difficile), E coli, klebsiella and enterobacter.[15] Prebiotics have been shown to be helpful with IBS (and particularly with bloating and flatulence.[16]

When you first start taking a prebiotic you can actually experience more flatulence and think that the prebiotic is making the symptom worse. But bear with it for around two weeks because once the levels of the good bacterial strains are increased the flatulence will subside. (The increased flatulence actually proves that the prebiotic is working.)

If you choose to take both a probiotic and a prebiotic, it is much better to take one supplement that includes both as they have a synergistic effect when taken together.[17]

CASE STUDY: ISLA

Isla was twenty-four years old and had IBS, recurrent thrush and was prone to stomach upsets, diarrhoea, difficulty in digesting fatty foods, bloating, wind and anal irritation. Isla struggles to eat large meals and can end up looking four months pregnant. Her stool test results showed that she had none of the beneficial bacteria lactobacillus, and two different negative bacteria as well as a parasite.

Isla was put on a gluten-free diet and given a programme of supplements to help eliminate the negative bacteria and parasite, a probiotic to take orally and also one that could be used vaginally, and a supplement to strengthen her immune function.

At her next appointment she felt a lot better and really liked the probiotic as she felt it calmed down her bowels. Her diarrhoea had gone but she still had quite a lot of wind so her programme of supplements was changed to focus on the flatulence, which she found very helpful.

GLUTAMINE

This amino acid is especially important for your digestive health as it is needed for healthy gastrointestinal function. It helps to maintain your gut barrier and heal leaky gut (see page 50) by nourishing the mucosal lining. It also has cleansing properties within the gut.

If you take it already combined in your probiotic then wonderful, otherwise you should take it separately – 50mg a day.

GAMMA ORYZANOL

This is a nutrient made from rice bran oil that helps to soothe your gastrointestinal tract. It helps to control the mini-inflammatory process that can be happening in your bowel and also seems to reduce the 'nervous' activity within the intestines.[18] Again it is helpful if the gamma oryzanol is in your probiotic to save you taking an extra supplement, otherwise take 50mg a day.

SACCHAROMYCES BOULARDII

Probiotic bacteria are the friendly bacteria that should be living in good numbers in your gut. However, there is also a probiotic yeast called saccharomyces boulardii which has been used to treat IBS.[19]

Taking a yeast supplement might seem a bit illogical in that you would think it could cause more problems with bloating and flatulence but saccharomyces boulardii is an interesting yeast. It manages to survive all the way through your digestive system, even through the very acid environment in your stomach, and is not wiped out by antibiotics as the good bacteria are. It helps with the growth of beneficial bacteria, so reduces inflammation in your digestive tract, and helps ward off negative bacteria. Saccharomyces boulardii has been used very successfully for helping with acute infectious diarrhoea, where it can reduce the duration by twenty-four hours.[20] This probiotic yeast has been shown to help with IBS,[21] and to improve the quality of life for IBS sufferers.[22]

Saccharomyces boulardii is thought to help with IBS because it increases the levels of an antibody called secretory IgA. Secretory IgA is found in mucous secretions in the gut and is your first line of defence against bacteria, yeasts and problem foods. If you are not producing enough secretory IgA then you are more susceptible to infections in the gut. You should take 400–500mg a day. (It is possible to test your level of secretory IgA – see page 52.)

DIGESTIVE ENZYMES

Digestive enzymes help to break down your food into smaller particles to make it easier for your body to use. The main digestive enzymes are:

- Lipases – these digest fats in the food you eat
- Amylases – these break down carbohydrates into simple sugars
- Proteases – these break down protein into amino acids

Common IBS symptoms can sometimes be caused by not having enough of these digestive enzymes, as food that is not digested efficiently can result in bloating and flatulence. The undigested food can ferment and give you a number of symptoms as well as being an ideal breeding ground for yeasts and negative bacteria. Digestive enzymes are taken with each meal so that they help to breakdown your food more efficiently. I would suggest you try them if you feel uncomfortable after eating. For some people this can occur after the evening meal when the meal is usually larger and you can be tired and your body (and your digestive system) is slowing down, in which case you would just take the digestive enzymes with the evening meal. You can buy good-quality digestive enzyme supplements from health food shops and you should take them as directed on the container.

Note: Do not take digestive enzymes if you have been diagnosed with gastritis, colitis or any ulcerative problem with the digestive system.

GINGER

Ginger has been used around the world for many years and is often found in Japanese, Indian and South Asian dishes. As well as being used in food it is often drunk as a tea.

It is often used to help with nausea, morning sickness during pregnancy and also motion sickness. It has a number of benefits for IBS in that it can help to prevent indigestion, gas and bloating. Ginger also acts as an anti-spasmodic and it relaxes and soothes your intestinal tract. It is also known to reduce anxiety, which for some people can worsen gastrointestinal symptoms, and contains a number of substances which can bind to the serotonin receptors in your digestive system in order to lessen some of the IBS symptoms.[23]

Ginger can be taken either as a tea or in supplement form. To get the maximum benefit, grate fresh ginger and pour on hot water, rather than using a ginger tea bag.

SLIPPERY ELM

This herb is native to North America and has been used for many years by the Native Americans. It helps calm and soothe the digestive tract by coating the lining of the intestines to reduce irritation and to calm the inflamed mucous membranes in the intestines. Slippery elm has this calming and soothing effect because it contains mucilage, which becomes a gel when combined with water.

Slippery elm is good for both constipation and diarrhoea as it can add bulk to stools if you have diarrhoea and soften the stools if you are constipated.[24]

Slippery elm can be taken either as a powder mixed with water or in supplement form. You should take 120mg a day.

MARSHMALLOW

No, not the soft sweets that come in pink and white, but a herb that has been used for over 2,000 years to help soothe and soften tissue. It has been used both as a food and also made into a poultice to be used to reduce skin inflammation. Like slippery elm it contains mucilage, which can reduce irritation in the digestive system and form a protective coating over irritated and inflamed intestinal mucosal membranes.

Marshmallow is taken in supplement form.

LICORICE

Licorice (also spelt liquorice) is a plant which is classed as a legume (the same as peas and beans such as soya) and the licorice extract can be made into sweets.

It can help to heal the irritated surfaces of your intestines and also has an anti-spasmodic effect, so lessening abdominal cramps. Licorice has been shown to help with IBS, especially when combined with slippery elm.[25] Too much licorice can increase the risk of high blood pressure because it causes the retention of sodium but there is a version of licorice called deglycyrrhized licorice, where the compound that causes the increase in blood pressure has been removed. So opt for a deglycyrrhized licorice supplement if you are taking it for a couple of months.

NOTE: Always speak to your doctor before taking any herbs. Because both slippery elm and marshmallow can coat the digestive system they may interfere with the absorption of drugs so it better to take these herbs away from medication.

CHAMOMILE

This is most commonly taken as a tea, especially in the evening or just before bed as it has a calming, relaxing effect on both the mind and body. And it is this calming and relaxing effect which is so valuable for IBS. It can reduce spasms and control 'nervous' reactions in the gut, making it less sensitive to food and other triggers. It also has an anti-inflammatory effect and can improve peristalsis (the muscular movement of the stool through your intestines).

FENNEL

Another herb which is often used as a tea, it helps prevent and relieve flatulence, as well as soothing the digestive tract and reducing cramps and spasms. You can also use it in your meals as part of your daily diet.

PEPPERMINT

Peppemint is a popular tea often drunk after a meal to help soothe and settle the digestive system. This herb has had the most research in terms of its effectiveness for reducing IBS symptoms. It can eliminate or reduce spasms, bloating, trapped wind, constipation and diarrhoea.[26]

TURMERIC

A spice used most commonly in Asian food that gives the food a bright yellow colour. It has significant anti-inflammatory effects throughout your body and has been shown to help 66 per cent of sufferers relieve the symptoms of IBS.[27] This can be used as a spice in cooking but it is more commonly used in supplement form, which gives you a higher dosage and is easier to take.

ARTICHOKE

Artichokes are eaten as a vegetable in many countries around the world. This vegetable, used as a leaf extract, has been shown to reduce the symptoms of IBS by over 25 per cent. People using the extract showed a significant shift away from bowel movements that were alternating between constipation and diarrhoea to a more normal pattern. There was also a 20 per cent increase in how they rated their quality of life. Interestingly the people in this trial not only had IBS but also dyspepsia (indigestion) and the artichoke helped to reduce this by up to 41 per cent.[28] Artichoke also acts as a prebiotic food by helping to 'feed' beneficial bacteria in the digestive tract.

A good combination supplement I use in the clinic containing peppermint oil, marshmallow, slippery elm, ginger, fennel, chamomile, licorice (deglycyrrhized) and artichoke is NHP's IB Support (BWL Support), available from health food shops or www.natural healthpractice.com.

ALOE VERA

Aloe vera is a succulent plant that grows in many countries around the world, often known for its ability to heal wounds and burns. It is thought to heal and soothe the digestive tract and so would seem to be ideal for IBS. But as yet there have been no clinical trials showing that aloe vera may help with IBS.[29] In my experience, some patients have found aloe vera juice helpful with IBS and others not, so it would need to be one of those herbs you need to try to see whether it works for you or not. But you need to make sure that you buy a really good quality aloe vera juice (which is made from the gel) or take it in capsule form. If you take the gel you do not want it to contain a preservative like sodium benzoate or benzoic acid – there are concerns that sodium benzoate may damage and inactivate DNA, which causes the cells to malfunction. This kind of malfunctioning could lead to premature ageing and general degenerative diseases.[30]

FIBRE

Taking additional fibre can also be very helpful for controlling IBS symptoms such as constipation and diarrhoea (which might surprise you). Fibre such as psyllium tends to be particularly helpful. Psyllium is adaptogenic fibre, meaning if you're constipated it will soften your stool and help increase your bowel frequency, and if you have loose stools and frequent bowel movements, it will help with stool formation and decrease the frequency of bowel movements. If you decide to use psyllium, make sure it is organic, as nearly all the products out there are not, and the damage from the pesticide residue in most of the products far outweighs the benefit you would receive from the fibre itself.

Another good fibre is whole, organic flaxseed. I suggest taking a few tablespoons of freshly ground flaxseeds per day. Another benefit of flax is that it's also a high-quality source of plant-based Omega 3 fats, particularly ALA, which nearly everyone needs on a regular basis.

FLUORIDE AND IBS

This is a very interesting topic because it carries with it some conflicting evidence but is an area that I think should be discussed.

A number of years ago, a study in Holland suggested that drinking water that was fluoridated caused gastrointestinal symptoms.[31] In a double-blind trial, the researcher showed that some people's gastrointestinal symptoms improved when they were drinking distilled water and returned when the fluoridated water was introduced. Other research has also shown that fluoride might cause nausea, vomiting and abdominal pain, all symptoms of IBS.[32]

Later research has shown a link between fluoride and indigestion,[33] and there are concerns that it could damage the lining of the digestive tract, which could lead to leaky gut (see page 50) and increased reactions to foods.[34] In the US, they say there are a few reports of gastrointestinal problems in people exposed to fluoridated water but suggest this is because those people are hypersensitive because of their IBS.[35]

In the UK, the Medical Research Council acknowledges the irritating effects of fluoride in relation to the stomach but states that 'it is possible that individuals who have an existing stomach disorder may be susceptible to irritation following ingestion of fluoridated water, but there is no published evidence for this. This issue is considered to be of low priority for further research.'[36] And that is one of the major problems; since this early research in the 1990s, and before that, there have been no studies on the effects of fluoride on gastrointestinal symptoms. And much of the past research on fluoride has 'failed to rigorously test for changes in gastrointestinal symptoms'.[37]

While there might not yet be conclusive evidence to suggest a link, this is one of those cases where you may want to test things out for yourself, perhaps reduce the amount of fluoride you are exposed to and just see if you feel any better as a result.

Only a small amount of the water in the UK is fluoridated but in the Republic of Ireland, for example, it is added to the water supply. If you are not sure you can ask your local water board to check the fluoride level in your tap water (if you have a problem getting this done, then get in touch with my clinic as we can organize this – see page 207). If your water is fluoridated the only water filter that can remove it is one that works on reverse osmosis. You can have this filter fitted underneath your sink in the kitchen for drinking and cooking water. The disadvantage of reverse osmosis is that it not only removes the fluoride but also valuable minerals like calcium and magnesium, however this may be a small price to pay (and you could then take a multivitamin and mineral to cover the lost minerals). Water can also naturally contain fluoride as it is derived from the minerals the water passes through – the level will vary depending on the source of the water.

The level of fluoride in your body can be measured with a simple urine sample so if you are concerned about this then do get in touch with my clinic for this test to be organized (see page 207).

Tips for reducing your exposure to fluoride:
Have your water tested to see if it is fluoridated (or ask your local water board if it is) and if so get a reverse osmosis water filter. When water is fluoridated in the UK it is about 1ppm

(part per million), in the US it can be up to 1.2ppm but recent guidelines are suggesting it has been lowered to 0.7ppm because of the risk of fluorosis (where the teeth become mottled with stains and pits in the enamel).

Buy fluoride-free toothpaste, as this is most likely your highest exposure to fluoride, especially if you swallow the toothpaste. Levels in toothpaste can reach as high as 1,450ppm in the UK, in the US it is lower – up to 1,100ppm. Fluoride-free toothpaste is readily available from most health food shops. (I would also suggest that when you are buying toothpaste you get a brand without sodium lauryl sulphate in it, as this can cause mouth ulcers and if it irritates the lining of your mouth, then perhaps it could also irritate the rest of your digestive tract.)[38]

Eliminate regular tea in all its forms, including black, green, white and red bush tea, as tea naturally contains fluoride. Herbal teas like peppermint and chamomile are fine.

Be aware if you are taking the antidepressant fluoxetine (also known as Prozac) that the active ingredient fluoxetine hydrochloride contains fluoride. Also statins, used to lower cholesterol, are fluoride based.

Don't use non-stick pans. The most common non-stick coating is made with fluorinated polymers and could increase the fluoride content of your food. If you are using non-stick then to reduce the risk of the non-stick coating eroding or flaking into your food avoid using abrasive cleaners, metal scourers or metal utensils when cleaning them.

NATURAL REMEDIES FOR CONSTIPATION

You may want some help getting your bowels moving while you are putting my dietary recommendations into place, but you don't want to take conventional laxatives. There are a number of choices available, and I will group them by the different ways in which they work.

STIMULANT LAXATIVES

As mentioned on page 36, these are not usually ideal for IBS sufferers as they can make symptoms worse. You could substitute the word 'irritant' for 'stimulant' as that is how they work and your bowel is irritable enough without adding to it.

Senna is a 'natural' laxative but is quite harsh. Another natural stimulant laxative is cascara, which stimulates the muscles in the intestinal wall to contract. Cascara will give you fast relief from constipation but you have to be careful that your body does not become dependent on it to 'go'. If you want to try cascara it is better to have it mixed in with other herbs such as barberry, ginger and wild yam to make the effect gentler but still effective. Cascara is taken in supplement form, usually along with other herbs.

BULK-FORMING LAXATIVES

These kinds of laxatives are mostly natural anyway as they are supplements of plant fibre. I would suggest that you try the psyllium husks (ispaghula) rather than bran, which is quite harsh and ironically can increase IBS symptoms. You can get psyllium husks in capsule form or in powder and they are just as effective taken either way but should always be swallowed with a good amount of water to help the bowel motion move easily along.

OSMOTIC LAXATIVES

These kinds of laxative work by drawing water into the stools to make them softer. These can include sorbitol and lactulose. Sorbitol is often used in diabetic foods as a sweetener but its side effect is diarrhoea. Sorbitol is found naturally in certain fruits such as apples, pears, peaches and cherries and is in higher levels in dried fruits like raisins and prunes, so to get a natural osmotic laxative you could use prune juice. As well as loosening up the stools it can cause flatulence as a side effect, so as with all of these remedies, see what works best for your body.

NATURAL REMEDIES FOR DIARRHOEA

There are some good natural remedies for diarrhoea but these should be used only in the short term while you are investigating the cause because, ultimately, the aim is to prevent diarrhoea in the first place, rather than just treat the symptoms.

Good natural remedies for diarrhoea are slippery elm and marshmallow (see page 137) – you can take slippery elm on its own but it seems to more effective with marshmallow. It can be taken in capsule form, as a tea, or the powder can be mashed up with banana and eaten as a paste.

The juice of grated ginger added to a cup of boiling water can be useful for diarrhoea when drunk every hour and so can carob powder when mixed with puréed apple (the apple contains pectin which can help to bind the stools). Fenugreek seeds added to water have also been used as a traditional remedy for diarrhoea. Use half a teaspoon of seeds and grind with 180ml hot water, leave for about five minutes and then drink the mixture.

ANTI-SPASMODICS

The aim with an anti-spasmodic is to relax the bowel to stop cramping and pain. So, certain herbal teas such as chamomile and ginger can be helpful with this. I have mentioned magnesium on page 128 because this helps with the relaxation of muscles and the bowel is a muscle that contracts to move the stool along (peristalsis). As well as taking magnesium as a supplement you can use magnesium as magnesium sulphate (Epsom salts) or magnesium chloride in the bath to help with cramps and pain. The magnesium is absorbed through the skin, hence the relaxing effect on muscles in general. Alternatively, you can spray magnesium oil directly onto your abdomen for relief.

This relaxant effect of magnesium is also useful for women who have painful periods, because the womb is a muscle, and it can also be helpful for other conditions like fibromyalgia, where muscles are affected. Magnesium can help reduce inflammation so may be useful for people with arthritis and general aches and pains. Magnesium

BODY BRUSHING

Before you bathe or shower take a natural bristled brush, ideally with a long handle, and brush your skin for a couple of minutes. Start with the soles of your feet and brush up each leg. Then from your hands along your arms to your shoulders. Brush upwards on the buttocks and lower back. You may prefer to not brush your abdomen, if you do use very gently strokes towards the centre.

Finally brush from the back of the neck to the front and very gently on the chest towards the heart, but not on the breasts. Don't brush your face or anywhere that feels tender.

baths or oil can also be helpful for skin problems such as eczema and psoriasis as it can reduce inflammation in the skin.

For a regular bath use one to two cups of magnesium salts in water temperature that is comfortable (not too hot). You could also try dry body brushing before you get in the bath as this will help to open up the pores to increase the absorption of the magnesium salts. A magnesium salt bath is best at the end of the day because you can just dry yourself off and get into bed afterwards (it is better not to rinse off the salts).

ANTIDEPRESSANTS

You may be reluctant to go on a prescription antidepressant for IBS symptoms when you are not actually depressed, even if you are feeling low because the IBS symptoms are getting you down.

The main herbal remedies that might be useful for depression are St John's wort and rhodiola. St John's wort (Hypericum perforatum) has been used for centuries and grows in Europe, Asia and America. It is classed as a weed and has yellow flowers. The small red dots on the petals contain hypericin, a compound that scientists believe is one of the active ingredients responsible for helping depression.

Over the past few years interest in this herb as a botanical anti-depressant has been enormous. It has been very well researched and the gold standard of reviews, a Cochrane review, of twenty-nine trials (including over 5,000 patients) stated that St John's wort supplements 'are superior to placebo in patients with major depression; are similarly effective as standard antidepressants and have fewer side effects than standard antidepressants'.[39]

Note: If you are already taking any medication, such as anti-depressants, you need to speak to your doctor before starting

TIPS FOR CHOOSING FOOD SUPPLEMENTS

- Read the labels carefully and avoid minerals in the form of oxides, sulphates and carbonates, as these are more difficult for your body to absorb. For example, you will absorb only an estimated 6 per cent magnesium when the mineral is in the form of magnesium oxide compared to 90 per cent magnesium when it is magnesium citrate.
- Choose minerals in the form of citrates (for example calcium citrate), which are more easily absorbed by the body.
- Choose a natural form of vitamin E (labelled d-alpha-tocopherol) rather than the synthetic version (Dl-alpha-tocopherol).
- Vitamin B6 as pyridoxal-5-phosphate is easier for your body to use than the cheaper pyridoxine.
- Look for vitamin D as D3 (cholecalciferol), which is 87 per cent more effective in raising and maintaining vitamin D levels than the cheaper D2 (ergocalciferol).[40]
- Choose a brand of vitamin C that says magnesium ascorbate (more alkaline than the acidic ascorbic acid and so better for IBS and for general health).
- When choosing fish oils, check both the EPA and DHA levels on the label and aim for 770mg EPA and 510mg DHA per day. Avoid cod liver oils as the liver is where the fish processes all of its toxins.
- Avoid probiotic drinks as they can be high in sugar. Instead, go for a supplement that does not contain maltodextrin (it's high GI and can affect blood sugar levels) and contains at least 22 billion organisms (including both lactobacillus and bifidobacteria strains). It's easier if you find one that is freeze dried as it won't need refrigerating so you can take it with you when you travel.

St John's wort. It has been suggested that it can stop the contraceptive pill from working properly and there are concerns about interactions with other drugs, such as those for heart problems, blood clots, epilepsy, migraines and also drugs after organ transplant and for HIV treatment.

Like St John's wort, rhodiola is thought to work by optimizing levels of serotonin in the body (as the SSRIs or Selective Serotonin Reactive Inhibitor drugs do). Rhodiola grows in cold climates and has been used in Russia for centuries. In one study it has been shown to significantly improve depression compared to a placebo,[41] and has been used to help combat fatigue, boost energy, improve memory.[42] It has also been found to reduce stress.[43]

OTHER NATURAL TREATMENTS

Other natural treatments such as acupuncture, homeopathy, osteopathy and reflexology can be extremely helpful for IBS and digestive problems in general and they can be used together with the nutritional and herbal recommendations in this book. A gold standard Cochrane review of the acupuncture studies on IBS has shown that it produced greater benefits than antispasmodic drugs.[44]

With homeopathy it is preferable to have an individual consultation with a homeopath but remedies such as argentum nitricum, asafoetida, lycopodium and nux vomica are often used for IBS and general digestive problems. Different aromatherapy oils can be helpful with IBS, including juniper, lavender, grapefruit and chamomile (see page 162).

As you can see from this chapter, nature offers us many ways to soothe and heal the gut. Just as with the medical options and with diet, the key is discovering what works for your body and also to be patient, as it can take time for any IBS treatment to really feel like it is making a difference. Some supplements work better for some people – aloe vera can feel very soothing for one person and make no noticeable difference at all for another. That's why I recommend the basic but essential programme of a good multivitamin and mineral, vitamin C and Omega 3 fish oils for everyone, and then build from there.

Supplements not only help with the healing process but also help your body to strengthen the gut and build a stronger foundation for your digestion. This is helpful, as once you have regained normal function you will be less likely to be affected by symptoms so easily. Combined with a healthy diet and lifestyle, you will begin to prevent symptoms from recurring and be able to relax and enjoy all those things that used to fill you with anxiety.

CHAPTER 7

STRESS, EMOTIONS AND EXERCISE

Of course it is vital to look at the physical causes of IBS and to address these using diet, supplements and medical treatments, but it is also important to look at the psychological side too. Your mind and body are very much interconnected and this is particularly the case when it comes to the digestive system, as it is so sensitive and responsive to your feelings and emotions.

As I explained earlier in the book, scientists talk about us having two 'brains', one located in our heads and the other in our gut where we have a nervous system (called the enteric nervous system) located in the sheaths of tissue lining the oesophagus (food tube), stomach, small intestines and colon. You have more nerve cells in your gut than you do in your spinal cord. This nervous system in your digestive system responds to emotions and stress in the same way as the brain, and its tissue is filled with the same neurotransmitters. Scientists talk about the 'brain-gut axis' because it is as though there is a direct line between the two and the messages can go either way – brain to gut or gut to brain.

It is thought that we ended up with these 'two brains' from evolution when we were just simple organisms that existed to eat and reproduce, and the nervous system of this simple animal was located in the gut. As we evolved with higher functions, a central nervous system was developed but the other one was left in the gut.

The way you think and feel can upset your gut but it also means that how your gut reacts to things can also affect how you think and feel. The best approach, therefore, is to tackle this from both sides at the same time. In Chapter 5 and Chapter 6 we focused on diet, nutrition and other natural remedies. Now, by looking at the emotional side alongside and putting in place some strategies to help calm your emotions I hope you will see an additionally positive effect on how your bowel functions and behaves. Gradually you will start to create a healthy cycle rather than a negative vicious cycle, which has kept you trapped by your symptoms and anxiety in the past.

THE STRESS AND IBS CONNECTION

If you feel that stress might be playing a large part in your IBS then this chapter is important for you. Feeling stressed and anxious can cause IBS because at times of stress the body needs extra amounts of energy. The stress response was designed to enable you to either run or fight for your life, and so the natural flow of energy during these times is diverted away from the digestive system to your extremities, in order to give you the energy to run or fight. Your body literally shuts down your digestive function, the secretion of digestive enzymes is halted and the natural pushing movement of the muscles of the intestinal walls slows right down, hence the symptoms of indigestion. Constipation results, food stagnates and ferments (making you bloated and giving you gas) and is eventually expelled from the body through bouts of diarrhoea.

Also, when the stress hormones are released, your body has to assume that you could be injured or that an invader (such as a bacteria) may be attacking your body so it prepares for these possibilities. Your body goes on alert and your gut will start to produce substances that cause inflammation in order to help the body heal any injuries. If you cut yourself you know that your immune system will go into over-drive to repair your skin by causing tenderness, redness, irritation and even heat and swelling, depending on the injury, and will mobilize its defences to protect and repair that cut as soon as possible, but in order to do that, it creates inflammation. That is a good thing when you are cut or injured but you definitely don't want that inflammatory response to occur in your body day in, day out just because you are feeling stressed – and especially not in your gut.

The stress response not only increases inflammation but it also changes the delicate balance of beneficial bacteria in your gut, making it more likely for negative bacteria or yeasts (like candida) to overgrow. It can cause leaky gut (see page 50), making you more reactive to certain foods that you are eating and it will make it difficult for the cells within your gut wall to regenerate, making the gut even more leaky.[1]

This stress response will also make your muscles contract, ready for you to run or fight. Bear in mind that your intestines are also a muscle, which means the food can be trapped inside and you might feel painful contractions in your gut. These muscle contractions are also caused by an imbalance between calcium and magnesium, which is, again, why magnesium is so important for IBS. When stress hormones are released, your body assumes you are going to be injured, so it releases calcium from your bones to help your blood clot at the site of an injury. Once the calcium is released, however, if it is not used because you have not been cut, your body cannot return it easily to your bones and so it gets deposited into your muscles and other tissues like your joints. Within your muscles calcium is used to help contraction and magnesium is used for relaxation, so having too much calcium in the muscles (in your gut and elsewhere) can cause cramps and spasms.

We also know that a traumatic event, such as an accident or divorce, can increase the risk of IBS so it is worth looking at how you can control ongoing stress or the impact it has on your body when you already have IBS.[2] Unfortunately, women are much more susceptible to the effects of stress and this may go some way to explaining why IBS is more common in women. Women are often trying to keep everybody happy, they are the 'people pleasers' and have a strong inner critic about what other people may be thinking, not only concerning what they say and do but also how they look. Equally, some men and women may feel inferior, carry emotional burdens or resentments, or perhaps have a tendency to try and be a perfectionist, all of which can drive the IBS symptoms.

TEST YOUR STRESS

How can you tell how stressed you are? Some people are good at hiding it but the physical effects will still take their toll, even if you maintain an air of calm on the outside – a bit like the swan who seems to be gliding effortlessly through the water but is paddling like mad underneath. There is now a very good laboratory test to assess stress, where a sample of saliva is collected at home and then sent to the lab for them to analyse your level of cortisol (one of the stress hormones that is released alongside adrenaline – see page 56 for more information on this test).

There is also a simple tool called the Social Readjustment Rating Scale, which is used by psychologists to predict the likelihood that someone may suffer from a stress-related problem like depression or IBS.

Using the table below, total up your scores for events that have happened over the past year. If a particular event has happened to you more than once within the last twelve months, multiply the value by the number of occurrences.

SOCIAL READJUSTMENT RATING SCALE

Event	Rating
Death of a spouse	100
Divorce	73
Marital (or other major intimate relationship) separation	65
Prison term	63
Death of a close family member	63
Personal injury or illness	53
Buying or moving house	50
Getting married	50
Fired from work or made redundant	50
Caring for sick or elderly relative	47
Marital reconciliation	45
Change in health or behaviour of a family member	44
Pregnancy	40
Sexual difficulties	40
Gaining new family member through adoption or remarriage	39
Business changes	39
Change in financial state	38
Death of a close friend	37
Change of occupation	36
Increase in arguments with partner	35
Taking on a mortgage	35
Increase or decrease in responsibility at work	29
Son or daughter leaving home	29
Trouble with in-laws	29
Commuting	28
Spouse begins or stops work	26
Start or leave school/university	26
Change in living conditions	25
Change in personal habits	24
Trouble with boss	23
Change in working hours or conditions	20
Change in living conditions (e.g. building work)	20
Change in type and/or amount of recreation	19
Change in social activities	18
Major purchase (e.g. car)	17
Change in sleep quality	16
Change in number of family get-togethers	15
Holiday	13
Christmas	12
Minor violations of the law (e.g. speeding ticket)	11

If you scored 0–149, you have experienced a fairly low level of stressful events over the last year and psychologists would estimate you would have a 30 per cent chance of developing a stress-related illness.

If you scored 150–299, the number of stressful events you have experienced over the last year would give you a 50 per cent chance of having a stress-related illness.

If you scored over 300, you have been through quite a year and it is really important that you now think about taking care of yourself. From your score, it would be estimated that you would have an 80 per cent chance of becoming sick from a stress-related illness in the near future.

These are major stress events that can tip you over the edge from seemingly being able to hold everything together to not managing at all. But many of these things are out of your control, they are thrust upon you and you simply have to deal with them. Then there are the day-to-day events which can have just as much an effect on your digestive and general health as these major traumas. The signs that you are living with chronic stress are having these sorts of feelings:

- That there are not enough hours in the day – it is one long round of keeping the plates spinning so they don't all fall down at once.
- There is no time for 'me' – this often affects women, especially those of the 'sandwich' generation who are working, have children and also looking after elderly parents. And no matter where they are and who they are with, they feel guilty because they are not somewhere else. They are trying to please everybody and that is just not possible.
- You are using caffeine and/or alcohol to get you through the day and evening.

- Your appetite has changed; you are either craving or binge-ing on sweet foods, chocolate, cakes, bread or have lost your appetite and are missing meals.
- You have lost your sex drive.
- You are biting your nails or picking the skin around the nails – signs of the stress response
- You are grinding your teeth.
- You get irritated or angry really easily by silly things (top off the toothpaste, waiting in a queue) and your reaction when you look back on it later seems inappropriate.
- Rushing around all the time to fit everything in.
- You can't seem to delegate – nobody is going to do the job as well as you so you need to do it yourself.
- You can't say 'no'.
- Forgetting things and not being able to concentrate well, as you are trying to retain and do too much.
- Tired but wired – you're finding it hard to get to sleep because your brain will not turn off, even though you are physically exhausted.
- Getting to sleep and then waking up in the middle of the night about 3 or 4am and finding it difficult to get back to sleep again.

REDUCING STRESS AND THE EFFECTS ON YOUR IBS SYMPTOMS

So would reducing the stress in your life and how you cope with it reduce your IBS symptoms? The answer is definitely yes. Research has shown that learning how to relax gives not only short-term but also long-term benefits in significantly reducing IBS symptoms and improving quality of life for IBS sufferers.[3] Because IBS is a condition of the gut and digestion, it is easy to focus only on diet when trying to find both the cause and the treatment for it. We might even become so worried about food or over-controlling to the point where our food anxieties make the physical symptoms worse. So dealing with our stress, anxieties and emotions are extremely important when it comes to recognizing and being aware of triggers, and also in helping long term to alleviate and even prevent the symptoms of IBS.

Simply learning some relaxation techniques can make a real difference, and as well as learning to relax, other psychological therapies have been shown to be significantly helpful for IBS symptoms such as abdominal pain and bowel dysfunction.[4] There are quite a few choices available that I would encourage you to have a look at and see whether you are drawn to a particular therapy.

CBT

Cognitive Behaviour Therapy can be very effective in helping to change how you think and to alter old patterns of behaviour. So if, for example, you have become caught in a negative thought pattern such as associating travelling on the tube or a plane with symptoms of your IBS and feelings of anxiousness, this therapy teaches you how to take a step back and stop yourself from over-generalizing and always fearing the worst. CBT will help you recognize the negative thinking patterns that are making you depressed and anxious. It then helps you to become more mindful with whatever you are doing and to be more in the now, rather than thinking of all the hundreds of other things you need to get done in the next few hours. Ask your GP to refer you to a CBT therapist. There are also many accredited private CBT practitioners in the UK.

Research on women with IBS has shown that mindfulness training, which is a technique used in CBT, has a substantial benefit for IBS sufferers in reducing the symptoms and improving quality of life.[5]

Here are some mindfulness tips to calm your mind:

- Practise observing your thoughts and feelings without analysis, judgement or criticism. Over time you are able to 'feed' negative thoughts less and less and so break free from a pattern of constant worrying or anxiety.
- Take your focus away from your thoughts and simply focus on your breath to help bring you back into the present.
- Focus on your present activity, whether it's a task at work, enjoyment and awareness while eating a meal or even just doing the washing up.

Hypnotherapy

CBT involves working with your conscious mind whereas hypnotherapy works with your unconscious mind. It works on the premise that there are two states of consciousness – the conscious and the subconscious – which may be at odds with each other. The aim of hypnotherapy is to give you control back over your thoughts and behaviours.

Habits are stored in the unconscious area of your mind and the benefit of hypnotherapy is that it enables communication with the unconscious mind to make the needed behavioural and emotional changes.

There is a specific type of hypnotherapy for IBS called gut-directed hypnotherapy which aims to not only help your general emotional state but also your gut health and digestive function, and evidence does show that it works.[6] Gut-directed hypnotherapy, as the name implies, focuses on your digestive system. During a session you would be asked to think about generating comfort and warmth in your abdomen. The sessions also aim to help improve your self-esteem and confidence. You will learn self-help techniques to help you relax the muscles in your gut and to control the symptoms of pain and bloating, and also to control emotions and behaviours that can worsen the IBS symptoms. Research on hypnotherapy and IBS has shown that it can give continued relief for up to five years after the hypnosis treatment has stopped.[7]

Counselling

Counselling or any 'talking therapy' can help with IBS if you are aware that there are issues and patterns of behaviour that may have developed from when you were younger.

Stress connected with going to the toilet can often be a problem and can alter the frequency of your bowel motions. Problems may have started in school where it was embarrassing to pass a bowel motion which might be noisy and smelly. Maybe you didn't have time to go before leaving home in the morning or it seemed better to wait until you got home at night instead of going at school. But suppressing the urge to 'go' can cause the bowel to become sluggish and stop it working efficiently. The same thing can happen at work if you delay a bowel motion because it is not convenient to go at the time. Your bowels need a routine – this might sound a bit strange, but it's important to encourage good bowel habits. By talking through the issues that have led to the formation of bad habits in the past, it is possible to help your mind change them into good ones.

Or you may have issues about going to the toilet from your childhood that have never been resolved. You may have been punished if you didn't go or there may have been problems about toilet training and you ended up soiling your clothes with feelings of guilt or anxiety conditioned around passing a bowel motion. For some toddlers passing a stool can be a strange sensation and so they may try to delay the experience as long as possible. Or periods of constipation that were uncomfortable are now associated with a negative experience of passing a bowel motion.

Meditation

This is another approach that can help you manage stress and your emotions and can have a beneficial effect on your IBS symptoms.

Meditation has been tested with IBS sufferers who were taught a relaxation-response meditation technique and it was shown to give a significant improvement in flatulence, bloating and diarrhoea.[8] A follow-up study one year later showed that the benefits were still significant when people continued to meditate.[9]

Dr Herbert Benson, an American cardiologist who founded the Mind Associate Professor of Medicine at Harvard Medical School, pioneered this relaxation-response meditation technique, which can be followed in six easy steps.

1. Sit quietly in a comfortable position.
2. Close your eyes.
3. Relax all your muscles, beginning at your feet and progressing up to your face, keeping them relaxed.
4. Breathe through your nose. Become aware of your breathing. As you breathe out, say the word, ONE, silently to yourself. For example, breathe in . . . out, ONE, in . . . out, ONE and so on. Breathe easily and naturally.
5. Continue for ten to twenty minutes. You can open your eyes to check the time, but do not use an alarm. When you finish, sit quietly for several minutes, at first with your eyes closed and later with your eyes opened. Do not stand up for a few minutes.
6. Do not worry about whether you are successful in achieving a deep level of relaxation. Maintain a passive attitude and permit relaxation to occur at is own pace. When distracting thoughts occur, try to ignore them by not dwelling upon them and return to repeating 'ONE'. With practice, the response should come with little effort. Practise the technique once or twice daily, but not within two hours after any meal, since the digestive processes seem to interfere with the elicitation of the Relaxation Response.

Massage

Massage can be a great stress reliever, which of course can help your IBS symptoms. Having a massage given by a trained practitioner is obviously going to be the best choice but if time and/or finances are at a premium then you can perform a gentle massage on yourself.

A gentle abdominal massage can be particularly helpful. The idea is to apply gentle pressure in circular movements that follow the direction of your bowels. So you would start at the bottom of your right side and continue to just under your ribs, across your middle and down the left hand side. I would suggest you use essential oils which can have a therapeutic effect. Some good ones for IBS are juniper to ease bloating, lavender to help promote relaxation, grapefruit for constipation or chamomile to help with cramping or discomfort. Remember, essential oils must be diluted in a carrier oil first. For a massage, add fifteen drops of one or several of the oils to six teaspoons of sweet almond oil. You can also use the oils in your bath – just add five drops of one or more to your bathwater.

Nutritional Supplements

There are certain nutrients that can help your body deal with the effects of stress. They actually reduce the amount of stress hormones released and so improve how your body copes with stress. B vitamins and magnesium have been discussed on pages 127–8 and are important when you are under stress. The B vitamins are even called the 'stress' vitamins and are known to help your body cope with stress – in particular vitamin B5 (pantothenic acid), which is the most important vitamin for your adrenal glands. Under constant stress, your body's need for this vitamin increases as it uses B5 to make the stress hormones. Magnesium is 'nature's tranquillizer' and is so important in helping to calm you down.

If you need extra help with controlling stress physically then I would suggest you add:

- Siberian ginseng – this is the best herb for tackling stress and is known as an adaptogen herb as it has a balancing effect on hormones. Siberian ginseng is a calming herb and can help your body cope with stress.[10] Siberian ginseng should not be confused with Panax ginseng (also called Asian, Chinese or Korean), which can speed up the body.
- L-theanine – this is an amino acid which has a relaxing, calming effect on both the mind and body.[11]

(There is a supplement I use in the clinic called NHP Tranquil Woman Support, which contains all these nutrients – available from health food shops or www.naturalhealthpractice.com)

CASE STUDY: PAMELA

Pamela, sixty-two, came to one of my clinics with symptoms of extreme constipation and a very painful, distended stomach. She compared her bowel movements to rabbit droppings, being incredibly hard and dry. Pamela could go for up to a week without opening her bowels, which consequently worsened her bloating and pain.

Her IBS came on quite suddenly last year after a bout of stress and she knows that stress really does exacerbate her symptoms. She was referred for a colonoscopy, which came back clear, and was sent away with not a huge amount of help apart from being advised to take antidepressants.

My nutritionist recommended Pamela follow a gluten-free diet for a month and she was given menu planners with lots of suggestions, which she found very helpful. She was also put on a tailored programme of supplements which included a multivitamin and mineral containing stress supportive nutrients, Omega 3 fish oils, a good probiotic, magnesium to relax the bowel and glutamine to help heal the gut lining.

Within a month Pamela had seen considerable improvement and was opening her bowels daily with properly formed motions. She found the gluten-free diet easier to follow than she first thought and was happy to continue because of how good she was feeling. She had a couple of days with symptoms but because she was keeping a food diary it helped her identify what she had eaten to cause this. Pamela had 'experimented' with supplements in the past but never really got it right and hence became despondent. However, the new supplements suggested at the consultation became a part of her daily routine and she really felt the benefit of taking them.

Pamela felt confident enough to move forward for a couple of months on her own and then would review again with another consultation. She was advised to continue with everything as she had been doing plus to continue to keep a detailed food and symptom diary so she could identify any difficult areas and discuss them at her next appointment.

IBS AND SLEEP

Sleep is important for your general health because it is the time when your body can recharge its batteries and repair its cells. It is thought that sleep is important for the health of your nervous system because when people are sleep deprived they are often more susceptible to mood swings and hallucinations and can feel confused and anxious. Lack of sleep can cause your body to produce more of the stress hormones, which is not good news for IBS (see page 152).

Unfortunately, stress and lack of sleep can become a vicious cycle because the less sleep you have, the less able you are to cope physically and emotionally with the demand of everyday life and the more stressed you feel ('tired but wired'). This then makes it harder to get a good night's sleep and you can feel trapped in this never-ending cycle.

It takes a lot of energy to digest food well (think about how tired we get after a big meal) and so not getting enough or good-quality sleep can affect your digestion. There is also a change in energy and blood flow to your digestive system as you sleep. It should be a time of rest, and if you stay up too late then your digestive system is also denied the rest it needs. Having a large meal at the end of the day, close to bedtime, is also not a good idea because your digestive system should be winding down at this time, not struggling with a large meal.

Not getting enough sleep or good quality sleep can increase your appetite and trigger cravings for foods that are not healthy. And with this increase in appetite unfortunately comes weight gain. A large study of nearly 70,000 women conducted over sixteen years found that those who slept less than five hours a night gained more weight over time than those who slept for seven hours a night.[12]

Interesting research has shown that people who have IBS, indigestion and heartburn often have insomnia.[13] This same study also confirmed what we know about stress in that those who have a lot of stress in their lives are twice as likely to have IBS, heartburn and insomnia. And the more your sleep is disturbed, the more severe the IBS symptoms can be.[14]

I think this is a chicken and egg question, because stomach upsets will cause disturbed sleep, especially if you are in pain or need to visit the toilet, but we also know that lack of sleep can cause stomach upsets.

I've added some tips below in order to help you get back to having a good night's sleep. This is important because the more disturbed your sleep, the more sensitive you become, especially in the rectal area, with research showing that you can end up feeling the urge to go more than you should and to react to pain more.[15] And the effects of sleep problems do not take a long time to show up. In fact, you could have one bad night of sleep and the next day your IBS symptoms can immediately be much worse.[16]

TIPS FOR A GOOD NIGHT'S SLEEP

- Caffeine acts as a stimulant so avoid any drinks like coffee, tea, cola and hot chocolate, especially after midday. For some people even drinking one cup of coffee in the morning can keep them awake at night so see if you can gradually cut down as caffeine is usually best avoided full stop for IBS sufferers.
- A cup of camomile tea will calm and relax before going to bed.
- Eating little and often during the day helps to ensure that your blood sugar stays balanced and that your digestion isn't overstretched late in the day. This also prevents the adrenal glands from working too hard, so that cortisol production winds down in time for bed.
- Alcohol affects blood sugar levels and so is best avoided. It also blocks the natural process of tryptophan being transported to the brain, which is important as tryptophan is converted into serotonin, the body's calming neurotransmitter.
- It's best to exercise early in the day as many people find it hard to sleep after an evening exercise session. Vigorous activity can delay the release of melatonin, which runs our internal body clock.
- Nocturnal hypoglycaemia is when you tend to wake in the middle of the night – often abruptly and with palpitations. It can help to have a small snack of complex carbohydrates, such as an oat cake or rice cake, or half a slice of wheat or rye bread, about an hour before bed. Again this helps to keep your blood sugar balanced so that adrenaline isn't released at the wrong time during the night. I know I usually say not to eat late in the evening but this is only a very small amount of food and you should only need to do this for a short time, maybe two weeks, while you are stabilizing your blood sugar during the day.

- To aid relaxation, add a few drops of aromatherapy oils like bergamot, lavender, Roman chamomile or marjoram to a warm bath before bed, or put a few drops on your pillow. A gentle massage with the same oils will also help to encourage sleep. If you are using the oils for massage then add fifteen drops of one or several of the oils to six teaspoons of carrier oil, such as sweet almond.

- Herbs can be extremely helpful for sleep-related problems. Hops, valerian, passionflower and skullcap all work as gentle sedatives and can help you to overcome insomnia. Try not to rely on only one herb, but rotate among several, to ensure that you don't become overly dependent. (Note: do not use these herbs if you are taking sleeping tablets.)

- Keep to a sleep routine, if possible setting your alarm for the same time each morning. And if you feel the need to catch up on sleep at the weekends, it is better to go to bed earlier rather than sleep in.

- Write any 'to do' lists at least an hour before bed, so your mind won't be whirring as you go to sleep.

- Sex or masturbation can help you go to sleep by relaxing you, and releasing tension.

- Magnesium, known as 'nature's tranquillizer', is good for helping with sleep problems as well as your IBS symptoms. If you suffer from restless legs or cramps, take both magnesium and vitamin E.

- Try this relaxation exercise. Lying on your back work up from your toes and tense then release each part of your body, ending with your face. You can feel the contrast between tension and relaxation and your body will usually become more relaxed as a result.

- Another good relaxation technique is visualization. Imagine yourself on a beautiful beach with the warm sun on your skin, soft sand under your feet, blue sky, clear water and the fragrant scent of wonderful coloured flowers. Or anywhere you like that makes you feel good and calm. This is really helpful for switching off from the day.

- Avoid watching TV, checking your mobile phone or working on the computer for at least an hour before you go to bed so that you are not exposed to bright lights or stimulation. Light exposure before bed can suppress the release of the body clock hormone melatonin which helps you go to sleep. And keep your bedroom a relaxed and restful place, sending signals to your brain that it is time to wind down. Don't read in bed or watch TV; if you do need to read during the night then make sure you get up and sit in the living room.

If you do shift work then this can make it harder to keep to a routine. For those of you who are working through the night, you are eating at a time when your digestive system will have slowed down so it can be more difficult to digest and absorb your food efficiently. You may also be eating in a rush and may be on your own because even at home you are eating at different times to your family. There may also be the tendency to use stimulants such as coffee and colas to keep you awake but these are going to have such a negative effect on your IBS. If you are on a night shift then have your main meal of the day just before your shift starts and keep to the 'little and often' rule during the night. The hardest time is 3 to 4am because we naturally get a drop in body temperature at this time, and you can feel very tired. Make sure you have some healthy snacks with you with a bit more protein for this time of the night (see the meal plan on page 98). And when you get home have a small snack that is higher in carbohydrates, so a small bowl of porridge for example would be good before you go to sleep – but nothing too large or heavy.

If you are using sleeping tablets I do encourage you to see your doctor about weaning yourself off these and, at the same time, examine what it is you are eating and drinking that may be affecting your sleep. As you sleep, your body goes through different stages of sleep and these stages are important. For the first two-thirds of the night you will have both deep and light sleep and in the last third of the night you will only have light sleep. Throughout the night REM (rapid eye movement) sleep occurs every ninety minutes. Unfortunately, sleeping pills can affect how you go through these stages and can also make you feel drowsy the next day.

EXERCISE

Exercise is known to help with IBS and research has shown that it can help with many of the symptoms including pain, bloating, bowel habits and quality of life. The research shows that exercise can help with all three different types of IBS, diarrhoea, constipation and alternating.[17] Exercise also has a number of benefits for your general health including:

- Improves mood and depression
- Improves body shape and weight
- Builds healthy bones
- Reduces the risk of heart disease
- Lowers high blood pressure
- Reduces high cholesterol
- Lowers the risk of breast and colon cancer
- Reduces the risk of developing diabetes

It also helps reduce stress and anxiety, which is important in helping to reduce your IBS symptoms. Exercise causes the release of endorphins (your feel-good neurotransmitters), which is why it helps with mood and depression, but these same endorphins also help to block pain signals.

At least thirty minutes of exercise five times a week is recommended. Find an exercise that you enjoy otherwise you won't keep going with it. Yoga can be helpful for IBS for a couple of reasons. It can work as a stress-reliever at the same time as strengthening your body. The other benefit from yoga is that it includes breathing exercises and often when we are stressed we shallow breathe. This is the automatic response when we are in the fight-or-flight mode because our breathing becomes faster and shallower to get a good supply of oxygen to the brain. So when you shallow breathe your body thinks that your life is in danger and this can increase how stressed you feel.

The opposite to that is deep, belly breathing that comes from your diaphragm, and this is what you practise in yoga. When you deep breathe your body registers that your life is not in danger and switches off the stress response. So this is an instant way of changing how you feel quickly.

When you are feeling anxious and stressed ideally it would be good to sit down for ten to twenty minutes to do the relaxation response meditation. But if you are not in a situation where you can do that and/or you don't have the time, just focusing on your breath for even a few seconds is very worthwhile. Wherever you are, standing or sitting, take a few breaths in and out through your nose. As you breathe in, push your belly out (you can put your hands over your belly to feel them being pushed out), pause briefly, and then breathe out slowly through your nose. As you breathe out, let go of all the stress and tension that you are holding on to. Even doing this once can make a huge difference in the moment but repeat it up to ten times if you can.

SMOKING AND IBS

As well as thinking about what you eat and drink that may be triggering or exacerbating your IBS symptoms, you also need to think about any lifestyle factors.

We know that smoking can cause heartburn (see page 180) and indigestion (see page 178) but it can also be a factor in IBS.[18] It is the nicotine in the cigarettes that is the main culprit because it irritates and stimulates the digestive tract, causing pain, diarrhoea and abdominal cramping. Some people even use smoking to help them go to the toilet or a double whammy of a cup of coffee and a cigarette. But smoking can also make you feel nauseous, which can be one of the symptoms of IBS, because cigarettes contain not only nicotine but also a number of toxins that your body can struggle to cope with. Smoking can also increase symptoms of bloating and flatulence because you gulp in air when you smoke.

When people stop smoking they may often experience constipation, which is a good 'side effect' if you have the diarrhoea kind of IBS but doesn't seem so good if you are often constipated. But as you will see later on in this book, there are natural remedies to help with constipation so you don't have to resort to smoking to help you to go. Unfortunately the nicotine in patch, spray or gum replacements can still cause IBS symptoms. I would suggest that you either use willpower to stop or, if you need extra help, a therapy like acupuncture or hypnotherapy.

I do think it is important to address the emotional side of IBS, whether stress is a trigger for your symptoms, or your symptoms in turn make you so anxious that it affects how you go about your daily life. I hope that by reading this book you feel confident that you have a practical plan that you can trust, which then allows you to feel more relaxed – and this can only help with healing your gut. And don't feel embarrassed to talk to close friends or family about the condition; sharing this kind of problem can make a big difference to how you feel about it. It's so easy to get caught in a vicious circle with IBS but there are many ways now to get help, from CBT to help with lifelong patterns, mindfulness to bring you into the now a bit more or relaxation techniques to use in everyday situations. Alongside the Diet Plan and supplements, approaching IBS through both the physical and the mind can work extremely well, both in the short term and in helping to prevent symptoms from recurring throughout your life.

CHAPTER 8

COMMON DIGESTIVE PROBLEMS

I want to include in this chapter all the digestive symptoms that many people complain of that may not be full-blown IBS but can cause so much discomfort including bloating, flatulence, burping, indigestion, heartburn, constipation and diarrhoea. Equally, if you are an IBS sufferer, then it may be helpful to focus on the specific advice for your individual symptoms.

Day after day you may be plagued with irritating digestive symptoms which are not in themselves a medical problem per se but which affect the quality of your life and can also give you many other supposedly unrelated symptoms such as fatigue, lethargy, headaches, skin problems and mood swings. By changing your digestive function, you can alter how well your body not only absorbs and digests the food that you eat but also how well it clears out waste matter, toxins and hormones.

BLOATING

This is such a problem, particularly for women. You may feel fine when you wake up but as the day goes on you feel more and more uncomfortable, with your clothes feeling tighter and tighter. Bloating can be caused by wind (see below), overeating or eating too quickly, constipation, food intolerance, candida (yeast) overgrowth and water retention (especially for women around their period). To overcome it you can address each cause individually.

OVEREATING OR EATING TOO QUICKLY

First of all, make sure that you are chewing well because the health and efficiency of your digestive system can be dependent on what happens during the first part of digestion, which takes place in your mouth through the action of chewing. Chewing not only helps with the mechanical part of digestion by breaking down your food into smaller pieces before it is swallowed but it will also make you eat at a slower, healthier pace.

When you eat quickly you can often eat too much as well. Overloading your digestive system with too much food can cause bloating because it takes twenty minutes for your brain to register that you are full. When you eat more slowly you will automatically end up eating less food.

CONSTIPATION

Being constipated can also cause bloating because bacteria in the bowel ferments food as it moves along the digestive tract. The longer the food stays in there the more fermentation and bloating can take place. And this will cause not only bloating but can also cause flatulence. See below for remedies for constipation – if you address this your bloating may go away, too.

FOOD INTOLERANCE

Certain foods may cause bloating – these can include any of the beans (such as chickpeas, lentils, kidney beans) and some vegetables such as broccoli, Brussels sprouts, cauliflower, cabbage, onions and leeks. Limit the amount of fruit you have to just three portions of fruit a day and avoid fruit juice completely or have just one small glass. It is a good idea to follow my exclusion diet recommendations (see page 65), keep a food diary (see page 65) and make a note of what you have eaten in the hours leading up to when you feel most bloated.

CANDIDA AND YEAST

If you have a candida overgrowth then when the yeast comes into contact with sugar it will ferment and can cause bloating. There is a simple test for candida overgrowth (see page 52) and if you test positive this can be treated.

EXTRA TIPS FOR ELIMINATING BLOATING

- Avoid soft fizzy drinks and carbonated water as these can cause bloating.
- Eat less raw food. Cooking helps to break down food, making it easier to digest. Patients have told me they can get bloated even from eating raw lettuce, which seems such an innocuous food.
- Get moving. Even a quick ten-minute walk can relieve bloating as exercise helps gas pass through the digestive tract more quickly.

WATER RETENTION

The best tip for eliminating water retention is often simply to drink more water as it is a natural diuretic. When you limit your intake of water your body often senses a shortage and so retains whatever water you do have. You should aim for six to eight glasses a day.

If you are looking for a herbal remedy, dandelion is the herb of choice for water retention. It is a natural diuretic that also contains more vitamins and minerals than any other herb, is an excellent source of potassium and helps improve liver function, which is good for general health and detoxification. I always recommend dandelion over synthetic diuretics as it allows water to be released without losing vital nutrients at the same time. The dandelion leaves can be used as a tea or in supplement form.

Water retention is often linked to eating too much salt. The World Health Organization recommends that we do not eat more than 6g (one rounded teaspoon) of salt per day. But most people end up eating about 9g of salt per day because it is hidden in so many foods, and ironically many of these foods with hidden salt are aimed at the 'diet' market. If fat is reduced in a food product then salt, sugar or artificial sweeteners and flavourings are often added to make it palatable.

Try to reduce your salt intake by using salt sparingly in cooking and get out of the habit of adding it to your food at the table. Try using other 'seasonings' instead like herbs, garlic, lemon or tamari (wheat-free) soy sauce in moderation. And always read food labels. Lots of processed foods like those in tins, packets or ready meals are surprisingly high in salt. And if you are buying tinned tuna, for example, then choose brands packed in sunflower oil or spring water rather than brine.

FLATULENCE

This is also known as wind or gas and again is very common. What you may not realize is that it is very natural to produce gas and it is only a problem when it becomes excessive and/or is smelly. My patients tell me that having flatulence is very difficult socially because it is embarrassing if they experience it when they are out. One patient even avoided sexual relationships because her wind was excessive and very smelly, especially at night in bed.

Flatulence often goes together with bloating, but not always. Flatulence is caused by either swallowing air or by the bacteria in your digestive tract. The worse smelling gas produced by the bacteria in the bowel is hydrogen sulphide, which smells like bad eggs. Gas can get trapped, causing discomfort as it isn't getting released, and sometimes the gas is absorbed internally rather than passed out.

Follow all the suggestions for bloating in the previous paragraph as the two often go hand in hand. The only time there is bloating without flatulence is with water retention.

As well as the dietary recommendations, I would like to stress the importance of taking a good probiotic and also digestive enzymes to help with both flatulence and bloating (see pages 132 and 135). And a cup of chamomile tea after eating may help as it has gas-relieving properties.

As always, you should aim to treat the cause of the problem, but if flatulence is a big problem, then while you are tracking down the cause you might like to use a supplement of activated charcoal to control the gas. Activated charcoal absorbs the excess gas but is not absorbed into your body so it carries the gas (and the smell) out through the faeces in a more gentle way than usual. It could potentially interfere with any medication you might be taking so check with your doctor before using.

BURPING

Burping, also known as belching, is excess gas that is expelled out through your mouth rather than the bottom. If you eat or drink too quickly then you can swallow too much air and cause your stomach to swell. Burping removes the air.

You may find that you end up burping after social dining because speaking frequently while eating can make you can swallow more air than usual. The same thing can happen if you snack on the run, drink from a straw or drink a lot of fizzy, carbonated drinks.

Helpful tips to reduce burping include making sure you chew your food well, slow down your eating and drinking and keep your mouth shut as you chew to prevent swallowing excess air. Try not to drink with meals, even water. If you want something to drink then either drink half an hour before or half an hour after eating. Also try having fruit separately from other food – so eat it as a snack on its own rather than after a meal because when you consume fruit with other food there is more chance of it fermenting and causing burping.

INDIGESTION

Indigestion happens when your body struggles to break down food and digest it properly. It generally describes a discomfort or a burning feeling in the stomach, often accompanied by nausea, bloating, flatulence, cramps, constipation or diarrhoea. Indigestion may also cause heartburn (see below) due to stomach acid reflux, which can leave a bitter taste in the mouth and irritate the oesophagus.

Indigestion is often caused by unhealthy eating habits, such as excessive intake of certain stimulating foods and drinks, and also lifestyle factors that put extra stress on your digestive system, such as smoking or being overweight. Certain common medications can also irritate the stomach lining and cause indigestion. To get rid of your indigestion, take note of the following natural indigestion-beating tips:

- Drink plenty of fluids but not with your meals, as this will dilute the digestive juices and stop them working properly.
- Remember to chew your food slowly and thoroughly. Chewing is essential for the digestive process and can help prevent indigestion. (Chewing thoroughly also reduces the likelihood of overeating as it allows the brain to register when you are full – see page 174.)
- Look at your posture and try to eat with a straight back rather than slouching over. Your stomach is just under your ribcage so if you are compressed in the middle then it makes it harder for your stomach to churn up the food efficiently. This is important if you tend to eat dinner bending over to a low coffee table or eat your food on your lap. You need to be eating at a table so that you are not bending over too much and can sit up straight between mouthfuls.
- Avoid drinking too many alcoholic and caffeinated drinks, which are known to trigger indigestion. Keep to no more than one drink a day and one or two cups of tea or coffee a day – herbal teas are of course fine.
- Avoid high-fat foods like chips, cheese and fried foods.
- Avoid spicy foods, like curry, if they make your indigestion worse.
- If you feel very full after a meal, take a brisk twenty-minute walk afterwards to ease uncomfortable feelings of fullness and prevent indigestion.
- Stress is a trigger for digestive upsets so try deep breathing,

which can help relieve stress-related digestive problems (see Chapter 7).

- Avoid taking aspirin and ibuprofen (these can irritate the stomach lining) and if you must take them do so on a full stomach.
- Leave a couple of hours between eating and going to bed and try sleeping in a more upright position, propped up on a pillow, to ease digestion pain at night. This will lessen the pressure on the stomach and prevent its contents coming back to remind you of what you ate during the day.
- Try a cup of peppermint or fennel tea after eating to help settle your stomach.
- Consider taking digestive enzymes as a supplement (see page 135) as they may help with indigestion by stimulating the release of bile, which can help with the digestion of fats, especially in the upper part of the digestive tract.

Persistent indigestion or heartburn (see below) should never be ignored because it could be a sign of a more serious digestive disorder such as peptic ulcers (caused by helicobacter pylori – see page 54 for information about a simple breath test), gastritis, hiatus hernia, gallstones and stomach cancer.

HEARTBURN

Heartburn is also known as acid reflux, and occurs when a teaspoon or two of stomach 'juice', or stomach acid, backs up into the oesophagus, burning its tender lining, and it is often accompanied by a burning sensation in the upper abdomen, nausea and retching. Symptoms also include chest tightness and a feeling of warmth sweeping your throat. Heartburn can make your chest feel as if it is on fire.

For millions of people, heartburn is an unwelcome experience and sales of antacids to help them cope increase every year. It can cause deep ulcers, lead to narrowing or obstruction of the oesophagus and cause bleeding. A particularly painful case of heartburn can mimic the symptoms of a heart attack so doctors advise that you visit your doctor or an emergency room immediately if you experience this.

Heartburn can be caused by certain diet and lifestyle habits. A fatty diet, too much alcohol, smoking and even chocolates can weaken the muscle that controls the opening between your stomach and oesophagus, called the oesophageal sphincter. Being overweight, especially around the middle, and wearing tight clothing can also make this muscle work less efficiently.

Meal times and meal size play a part. If you eat a large meal quickly and then lie down you are asking for trouble. A full stomach puts pressure on the oesophageal sphincter and lying flat makes it easy for acid to flow backwards. Other causes include straining while coughing, constipation, aspirin and some prescription drugs.

If you are in a lot of pain and need quick relief a chewable or liquid antacid will do the trick but I don't recommend long-term use of antacids because they don't treat the underlying cause, which is most likely to be your diet and lifestyle habits. There is a natural alkalizing supplement (containing sodium bicarbonate) rather than a conventional antacid that I use in the clinic which is called Bio-carbonate, but it is still better to address the cause in order to get long-term relief.

If you would like to try some natural ways to soothe the pain I suggest you do the following:

- Choose foods carefully. Certain foods and drinks can make reflux worse and so they should be avoided. Foods that irritate the oesophagus and make the burning sensation worse include chocolate, foods rich in saturated and trans fats and coffee, both decaffeinated and regular. Citrus juices and fruits, tomatoes, tomato juice, spicy dishes and onions can also aggravate the problem for some people so they should be eaten with caution.

- Eat early. Sitting down to dinner at least three hours before you go to bed will ensure that your stomach isn't full when you go to sleep.

- Eat little and often. Aim for five or six meals and snacks a day instead of three big ones. There is less pressure to cause reflux this way.

- Lose excess weight. Even losing just a few pounds can significantly alleviate heartburn because extra weight around the middle can squeeze the oesophagus and stop it tightening as it should, which makes reflux worse.

- Quit smoking and cut down on alcohol. If you haven't already, quit smoking because smoking is a well-known cause of acid reflux. Alcohol can also make the sphincter muscle work inefficiently and irritate the oesophagus.

- Loosen your belt. Tight belts or waistbands can increase the pressure on the abdomen and make reflux worse.

- Lie on your left side. Studies show that if you must lie down after a meal it is better to lie down on your left side. Experts speculate that this is because lying on the right side puts the junction of the stomach and oesophagus lower than the gastric pool in the stomach, making it easier for acid to seep into the oesophagus.

- Try yoghurt. Milk is traditionally said to soothe heartburn but it is thought that it only gives temporary relief and then actually causes an increase in stomach acid, so making indigestion worse. Try milk in the form of yoghurt instead. A good home remedy is to mix a tablespoon of live yoghurt containing beneficial bacteria into a glass of water and drink it, or open up a probiotic supplement and mix that with water instead.

- Drink herbal teas. Peppermint, chamomile, slippery elm and ginger tea can also help.
- Eat papaya. This contains papain, an enzyme that can naturally soothe your stomach. But papaya is high on the FODMAP diet (see page 110) so could increase IBS symptoms. If you suspect papaya could affect you in this way, you can take the papain in supplement form instead.
- Remember a good tip to avoid heartburn and also for good digestion generally is 'don't dine after nine'.

CASE STUDY: MAUREEN

Maureen, aged fifty-two, came to one of my clinics for help with constant painful bloating, difficulty digesting fatty foods and reflux and a history of ulcerative colitis. She was given medication for the reflux but this made her feel sick so she was reluctant to take it. Maureen was keen to sort this out naturally rather than taking drugs to mask what was really going on. She herself had realized that wheat, caffeine and alcohol aggravated her symptoms so she tried to stay off them as much as possible, but found it hard to be consistent especially when she was stressed. Stress was a major part of her symptoms and she found it hard to manage, although wine did help, even though she knew it exacerbated her IBS.

During the consultation Maureen was given a more structured eating plan to follow, avoiding wheat and caffeine and alcohol. She was asked to drink aloe vera on a daily basis, which is naturally soothing on the gut and has been known to balance acidity. She felt motivated to start the programme because she had the support of a qualified nutritionist, whereas in the past she had started to try cutting food groups out but didn't have the impetus to keep at it.

Maureen was recommended some nutritional supplements to support her stress levels, including magnesium, Siberian ginseng and L-theanine. A good-quality probiotic was added to her programme together with fish oil for its anti-inflammatory effect. It was also suggested that she try to address her stress by incorporating some techniques like breathing exercises. She was asked to complete a daily food diary, making a note of her symptoms on a scale of one to ten, so she could discuss it at her next appointment.

At her follow-up appointment six weeks later, Maureen had shown marked improvement, with less bloating; scoring a two out of ten rather than 10. She followed the eating plan the best she could but work commitments made it difficult to stick to it 100 per cent. She felt eating wheat in moderation had much less impact on her body, which she was pleased about. She was finding the supplements really helpful, especially the stress-calming nutrients.

Overall Maureen was pleased with the outcome of the consultation and she felt that she understood her body a lot better now. She agreed to continue with the low-wheat, -caffeine and -alcohol plan and would be consistent with the supplements until the next review in eight weeks.

CONSTIPATION

Constipation is such a common 'condition' in our modern-day lives – we have less time to actually go to the toilet and our diets contain so much more processed, convenience foods and less fresh food.

You should be aiming to have a bowel motion every day. Toxins and waste products should be excreted via the bowels and if they are sitting there not being passed out, then the toxins can be reabsorbed back into the bloodstream. In the longer term this can lead to malabsorption of vital nutrients and will make you feel lethargic, sluggish and miserable. To make matters worse you can often experience painful bowel movements and an increased risk of haemorrhoids (piles) through straining. And for women, being constipated is associated with having more urinary tract symptoms such as increased frequency, urgency, infections, incontinence and nocturia (getting up frequently in the night to spend a penny) so it is critical to sort out constipation.[1]

Constipation can be caused by a number of factors including medication, hormonal changes in the menstrual cycle, not enough fluids, not enough exercise, stress and lack of time. Iron supplements are often a common cause of constipation because if your body cannot absorb all the iron from the supplement it gets excreted through your bowel causing your stools to become blacker and harder as the iron reduces the amount of water your stools are absorbing. The biggest culprit is iron in the form of ferrous sulphate, which is very difficult for your body to absorb and so more of it ends up being excreted through the bowel. There are more absorbable supplements of iron that do not upset your bowels; these forms include iron citrate and ferrous bisglycinate.

Unfortunately there is still a lot of confusion surrounding constipation and it is still widely recommended that a high-wheat-fibre and bran diet is consumed. But this is not the long-term answer as it can irritate your digestive system and actually cause bloating and give you irritable bowel-like symptoms.

TIPS FOR RELIEVING CONSTIPATION

One of the most important tips for helping with constipation is to increase your fluid intake. I know everyone talks about drinking six to eight glasses of water a day for our general health but this fluid intake is crucial if you are constipated. The fluid stops your stools becoming dry and hard and helps the waste to move along the bowel easily and comfortably.

The fluid does not have to be eight glasses of cold water a day. A cup of herbal tea counts as one of your eight glasses, or a glass of hot water with a slice of lemon first thing in the morning. Ordinary tea (rather than herb teas), coffee and alcohol will not count, however, as they are dehydrating. A healthy diet is also likely to contribute to the important eight glasses of liquid. When you eat a more healthy diet you will be including more watery foods naturally, such as fruits, vegetables, brown rice and soups, which all contribute to softening your stools and therefore relieve constipation.

I would suggest experimenting with your diet by eliminating wheat but you can include oats. Also eliminate all caffeinated drinks such as coffee, tea and colas. I know that some people use caffeine to help them go to the toilet because it acts as a stimulant. But this can irritate the digestive tract and over time can make bowel problems worse so I don't recommend it as a solution.

Don't put off going to the toilet and don't strain to rush a bowel movement. It is easy to think that time is short and leave the house in the morning without going. You need to retrain your bowel by getting into a daily routine of leaving time to go when you get up or after breakfast.

Sit and relax on the toilet and at first you may only pass urine or gas but over time the daily habit of sitting on the toilet at the same time can help release a bowel motion. Don't sit there for longer than fifteen minutes as any longer is not going to help. Also at any time when you feel the urge to go, go – don't postpone going, because your bowel will get lazy. The walls in your rectum expand as they fill with the stool and it is this stretching that gives you the message to go to the toilet. This message only lasts for a short period of time, about fifteen minutes, so it is possible to ignore it. But if you ignore this message to go then the rectal walls may have to fill up with a larger bowel motion in order for the urge to be registered. And the longer the stool sits in the bowel the more water is removed from it, making it harder to go the next time. Your bowel is a muscle and if you stop using a muscle then over time it stops working properly.

And that is the problem with using laxatives. Nature is very sensible – your body thinks, well, why do the work if something else is going to do it? So the more you use laxatives, the lazier your bowel can become. There are two kinds of laxatives: ones that stimulate and ones that have a bulk-forming action. It is the stimulating type, like senna, that can make your bowels lazy, so although they are tempting, I recommend you do not take these laxatives.

An excellent natural remedy for constipation is to soak one tablespoon (15ml) of whole flaxseeds (linseeds) in water for at least thirty minutes and swallow first thing in the morning or last thing at night (you need to experiment to see which time of day works for you, morning or night). The soaked linseeds form a mucilaginous substance that is moist and sticky and helps your stools to slip easily and smoothly through the bowel and out the other end. The flaxseeds act as a bulk-forming kind of laxative and are very mild so can even be used in the long term. But the aim is to make changes in your diet so that over time you may only need to use the flaxseeds every other day, then every two days and so on to the point where eventually you don't need to use them at all, because your bowels are functioning normally. Psyllium husks can also be used but I would suggest you try the flaxseeds first as they seem to be gentler.

The mineral magnesium in the form of magnesium citrate is also good for helping with constipation. It helps to increase water absorption in your intestines and improves peristalsis (the contractions that move your food along). Take a supplement of about 200mg with your evening meal and see what happens the next morning. If your stools are comfortable, then leave it at that amount, if not, take about 400mg the next evening and along with the dietary and supplement recommendations you are following, you should soon end up with an amount of magnesium citrate that gives you a comfortable stool. Over time you then want to see if you can reduce the amount of magnesium so that eventually you don't need to take any.

Vitamin C also can help with constipation and, as with magnesium, you should start off with a lower dose such as 500mg morning and evening and then increase by 500mg each day until your stools are soft and comfortable. I would suggest you use the alkaline form of vitamin C, magnesium ascorbate, and not ascorbic acid (see page 130 for more information about vitamin C supplements). Over time you should be able to reduce the vitamin C to a maintenance dose of 500mg twice a day. You can take both the magnesium citrate and vitamin C at the same time. It does not have to be one or the other.

A good probiotic supplement will help improve the levels of beneficial bacteria which in turn help with the peristalsis in the bowel (use a probiotic that contains at least 22 billion bacteria – a good one I use in the clinic is NHP's Advanced Probiotic Support, available from health foods shops or www.naturalhealthpractice.com).

I am often asked in the clinic whether having a colonic (also known as colonic hydrotherapy and colonic irrigation) is a good idea for help with constipation. If you have had chronic constipation then it would be worthwhile having a treatment as it uses warm water under very low pressure to flush out the colon. Choose a practitioner who is registered with an organization and is fully insured. Colonic hydrotherapy is not something that I would suggest you have on a regular basis, however, because as well as flushing waste it also depletes your body of the beneficial bacteria. Also some people have been known to get 'hooked' on the feeling of emptiness that the therapy can give and end up having one a week, which I would definitely not recommend.

Finally, if you suffer from constipation, make sure that you undertake regular exercise, as this helps to increase the muscle contractions in the bowel to move the stools along.

DIARRHOEA

The biggest problem with diarrhoea is that it causes the loss of certain nutrients called electrolytes such as sodium and potassium, which are important because your cells, especially in your heart and nerves, use them to carry electrical impulses. Sudden and acute diarrhoea can be caused by an infection picked up through food poisoning and if diarrhoea continues for more than three days or is bloody you should get it investigated.

If your diarrhoea is long term and you have been investigated for infections (and nothing was found) then it will be worth investigating if it is triggered by your diet. I would suggest you take out all the foods below for about a week and see what happens to your stools. If they are much improved then add in the foods again one at a time, to try to pinpoint the specific food causing the diarrhoea:

- Dairy – it might be the lactose that is the trigger or the high fat content
- High saturated fat foods like red meat, sausages
- Caffeinated drinks such as coffee, tea and colas – caffeine works as a stimulant and increases the natural contractions of the bowel so can move the stool faster through your body
- Citrus fruits – these may aggravate your digestive system
- Foods that contain sorbitol as a sweetener – this is often used in diabetic foods and one of its side effects is diarrhoea.

EXTRA TIPS
Address your stress levels (see Chapter 7) because feelings of anxiety and tension will be sensed by your digestive system and can increase the transit time of your stools through your bowel.

With diarrhoea you will be having an increased transit time, which means that your food is passing much faster through your digestive system than it should do. The problem with this is that it can make you deficient in a number of nutrients because you are not absorbing them through your food. I would suggest that you take a good multi-vitamin and mineral to help you stay healthy. Take a good probiotic (containing at least 22 billion organisms) as this will make sure that the balance of bacteria in your gut is good. (See page 126 for more on my recommended supplement programme.)

Antibiotics can give what is called medically 'antibiotic associated diarrhoea', in which the antibiotics cause diarrhoea by altering the balance of 'good' and 'bad' bacteria within the gut or by causing an overgrowth of candida. If you have had to take frequent doses of antibiotics in the past then take a probiotic for at least three months and see if this makes a difference to your diarrhoea. If you are on antibiotics at the moment then do still take a probiotic but take it at a different time of day from the antibiotic.

Good natural remedies for diarrhoea are slippery elm and marsh-mallow. These have been mentioned on page 137 and are particularly calming to your digestive system.

LEAKY GUT

Research has shown that leaky gut (see page 50) is often present if your IBS started after you had a gastrointestinal upset or food poisoning.[2] The risk of developing IBS after a gastrointestinal infection increases six fold and can remain high for up to three years after the infection.[3] It is thought that IBS that develops after an infection is caused by a combination of leaky gut, changes in the levels of beneficial bacteria and also persistent inflammation in the gut.[4] As well as a gastrointestinal

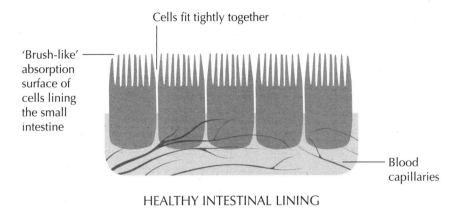

Cells fit tightly together

'Brush-like' absorption surface of cells lining the small intestine

Blood capillaries

HEALTHY INTESTINAL LINING

Gaps between cells are wider – partially digested food particles can slip through

Damaged absorption surface of cells lining the small intestine

Blood capillaries

LEAKY GUT

infection, leaky gut can be caused by antibiotics, NSAIDs like ibuprofen, candida (see page 153), too much alcohol or too much stress.

Symptoms of leaky gut are often the same as those of IBS and include:

- Bloating
- Flatulence
- Abdominal cramps
- Fatigue

- Joint pains
- Skin rashes
- Food sensitivities

I usually recommend that patients are tested for leaky gut if they present with IBS symptoms, as well as a stool test to measure their levels of bacteria, check for negative bacteria, parasites, yeast (candida) overgrowth and also measure levels of inflammation (see Chapter 4 for information on all of these tests).

WHY CANDIDA CAN CAUSE LEAKY GUT

Candida is a yeast which occurs naturally on the skin, in the mouth, vagina and digestive system. Depending on the circumstances it can overgrow, causing problems like thrush (vaginal yeast) and toenail infections.

Candida also resides in the intestines and under healthy circumstances is kept under control by the levels of your beneficial bacteria and your immune system. But if you are under stress or your immune system is not strong then the single-celled yeast form changes into a form which has roots. These roots (also called rhizoids) are able to pierce the walls of the digestive tract and break down the protective barriers between the intestines and the blood.

This 'breaking-through' the barrier allows the candida to invade your whole body causing an infection of this yeast, which is known as candidiasis. Symptoms of candidiasis include persistent vaginal thrush, bloating and flatulence, cravings for sugar and bread, getting tipsy on a small amount of alcohol, brain fog, athlete's foot and fungal toe as well as food sensitivities. It is better to test to make sure that you have candida (see page 51 for information on testing for candida). If you have candida you will need to do three things: follow an anti-candida diet (see page 51 for advice on this), re-colonize your gut with good bacteria and eliminate the candida overgrowth using natural remedies.

If you do the candida test by post, all this information is included and of course if you come into the clinic you will be given all the information you need to correct the candidiasis, and help with any health problems as well.

CASE STUDY: JANE

Jane, fifty-seven, has had IBS and stomach problems for over fifteen years. She was plagued with bloating, wind and a burning feeling in her stomach, was prone to stomach upsets and also had difficulty in digesting fatty foods. Jane was aware that her symptoms got worse when she was stressed and she would get stomach pains then too. She had dysentery in the past from travelling and used to get a lot of thrush and cystitis. Jane was also putting on weight and because she had bloating, too, her doctor had suggested that these symptoms were down to her age and the menopause.

Jane was already taking a probiotic and aloe vera juice when she came into the clinic. A stool test was recommended to check what was happening in her bowels. Her stool test results showed that she had good levels of bacteria (she was asked to stop the probiotic for three days before doing the test) but there were negative bacteria present. The stool test also indicated that Jane was struggling to absorb carbohydrates.

My nutritionist suggested Jane try eliminating gluten from her diet, avoid foods containing yeast and keep fruit to a minimum. She was also put on a programme of supplements including a probiotic, aloe vera juice, and a supplement containing a number of enzymes which help to digest the carbohydrates that yeast feeds off (so effectively starving the yeast), and also digest the protein nucleus of the yeast organism to gently remove it from her body.

By her fourth appointment, Jane was feeling much better, her bowels had improved considerably and she could eat normally without bloating and discomfort. She was still taking the supplements and following a gluten-free diet as much as she could.

At her last appointment Jane felt her bowels were so much better and she had hardly any symptoms at all.

'SIDE EFFECTS' OF HAVING IBS

Here I have included some of the common problems that are experienced as a consequence of having IBS. Not everyone with IBS will get these problems but if you do experience any of them, then know you are not alone and there is plenty you can do for relief.

PILES

If one of the major symptoms of your IBS is constipation then one of the consequences of that can be piles, also known as haemorrhoids. When you constantly strain to go to the toilet it puts pressure on surrounding veins and affects blood flow. Piles are varicose veins around the anus and rectum and under the pressure of straining the veins become wider and can become engorged with blood.

Piles can be inside and/or outside of the anus and can be large or small and will feel like lumps. Sometimes they can be painless and the only symptoms may be bleeding after you go to the toilet (any bleeding must be checked out though to rule out anything more serious). Some larger ones can cause pain and itching and there may also be a mucous discharge. For many people, piles can heal up and go away on their own, but usually once you have them you are likely to get them again.

All the dietary and supplement recommendations in this book are important for helping with piles because they will eliminate the constipation and the need to strain when going to the toilet. There are also over-the-counter creams readily available that can be used to ease any discomfort while you are getting the benefit from the changes in your diet.

As a natural remedy, witch hazel has traditionally been used to dab on the piles as it acts as an astringent.

DIVERTICULITIS

It is thought that when the muscles of the intestines are strained due to constipation that this pressure can cause bulging pouches (diverticuli) to develop in the lining of the intestines, which over time can become inflamed or infected. A diet too low in fibre is thought to be the main cause of diverticulitis. People can have diverticulitis without having IBS but they can be connected. Diagnosis of diverticulitis is done with a barium enema (where barium is inserted into the rectum and shows up the intestines on an X-ray) or a colonoscopy (where a camera is inserted into the anus to look at the intestines).

The nutritional recommendations you are following in this book can be helpful for diverticulitis (see Chapter 5) and if there is an infection you would probably be given antibiotics (I suggest you also take a probiotic to restore the good bacteria) or surgery to remove part of the intestines containing the diverticuli.

FAECAL INCONTINENCE

The opposite side to the problems connected with constipation is the consequence of having diarrhoea, which can lead to incontinence. There are two types of faecal incontinence, one in which someone has no feeling that they have been to the toilet, called 'passive incontinence', and one in which the person knows they need to go but can't get to the toilet in time, called 'urge incontinence'.

Again, follow all the dietary recommendations in this book (see Chapter 5) for diarrhoea and use the remedies like slippery elm (see page 137). It would also be worth taking some exercise classes such as Pilates to help strengthen your core abdominal muscles including the pelvic floor muscles.

Pelvic floor exercises (also known as Kegel exercises) which strengthen the pelvic floor can be especially useful for both men and women to prevent incontinence. There are two types of muscles that need to be worked, and two types of exercises to work them. First of all, slowly bring up your pelvic floor by contracting the muscles. Hold for a count of five and then gently let it down again. Work at this, several times a day, until you can hold the count for fifteen. You may find that you lose control part way through the count. Start again, and make sure that you can feel the muscles being released as you 'let down' your pelvic floor.

The second type of exercise involves quick tightening and releasing of the muscles in the pelvic floor. As quickly as you can, tighten and then release the muscles. Do this about thirty times, and then take a break.

Each session should comprise two sets of the 'slow' exercises and two sets of the 'fast' exercises. Take a minute's break in between. Some people find it easier to practise these exercises while sitting on a kitchen chair because you can actually feel the muscles as they rise and fall against the chair. In the beginning it may also help to perform the sets while lying down, because the pressure of gravity is reduced.

Instead of complete faecal incontinence you may experience something called anal leakage, where just a small amount of liquid bowel matter is passed out. This can be just as embarrassing as full incontinence and again it is important to put into place all the recommendations in this book. Ironically, anal leakage can happen with either the diarrhoea type of IBS or the constipation predominant type. With constipation, there can be a hard stool stuck in the rectum but liquid stool is leaking out around it.

Anal leakage can also happen when you think you are passing wind but a small amount of liquid bowel matter can pass out instead. The pressure of the flatulence seems to cause some of the faeces to pass out. Again you need to follow the recommendations in this book, because by treating the cause of the flatulence you can stop the leakage.

NUTRIENT DEFICIENCIES

As IBS affects the digestive system you may suffer from malabsorption of certain nutrients. This is often the case with iron and vitamin B12. And if you are having to avoid whole food groups to ease your symptoms then you may be missing out on other nutrients in order to prevent flare ups as you give your gut time to heal.

A deficiency of vitamin B12 can give you diarrhoea or constipation so it is important that you have a blood test to check for this vitamin just in case there is confusion over your symptoms. Other symptoms of a B12 deficiency include dizziness, fatigue, weight loss, irritability, weakness and tingling in the hands and feet.

Iron deficiency anaemia occurs when haemoglobin levels in the red blood cells are low. Because red blood cells provide oxygen to your tissues, tiredness can often be one of the major symptoms. Other symptoms can include shortness of breath, dizziness, sore tongue and headaches. When you are tested for anaemia, the lab measures the level of iron available in your red blood cells (haemoglobin). However, iron is also stored as ferritin in other parts of the body, such as the spleen and liver. When your doctor orders tests, make sure that both your haemoglobin and ferritin are checked, as it is possible to be iron deficient even if your haemoglobin levels are normal.

You can increase your iron intake by taking your iron tablet on an empty stomach and if you take it with a vitamin C supplement this can also help to improve absorption. To help your body absorb the iron from your food more efficiently, don't drink black tea fewer than thirty minutes before or after a meal as the tannin in the tea blocks your body's uptake of iron (and other minerals, such as calcium).

Avoid taking iron in the form of ferrous sulphate (also called iron sulphate), which is classed as 'inorganic' and is less easily absorbed by the body. Only 2–10 per cent of the iron from this type of iron supplement is actually absorbed by your body, and even then, half is eliminated, causing blackening of your stools and constipation. Organic irons are much more easily absorbed and do not affect your bowels in same way. Phosphates found in fizzy soft drinks also prevent iron from being absorbed by the body. Herb teas and fruit juices are fine.

You can increase your iron intake with food such as eggs, leafy dark-green vegetables, seaweed, apricots, millet and whole grains. I am not a fan of liver, however, as it is the most polluted part of an animal as all toxins and waste are dealt with by this organ.

GERD

GERD stands for gastroesophageal reflux disease and occurs when the sphincter at the bottom of the oesophagus (the food pipe) does not work properly and lets the contents of the stomach go back up, giving a burning sensation known as heartburn. I have covered heartburn on page 180 and it is important to know that it can go hand in hand with IBS, with nearly 80 per cent of IBS patients having symptoms of GERD. Nobody knows for sure why there is this connection but it could be that the whole digestive system is very 'irritable' and sensitive and this affects both the top and bottom half of the digestive tract.

OTHER CONDITIONS COMMON TO IBS SUFFERERS

In this section I will cover two other health problems, fibromyalgia and Chronic Fatigue Syndrome. Although they are not strictly speaking 'side effects' of IBS, they are conditions that often have IBS symptoms alongside so I felt it important to include them.

FIBROMYALGIA

Fibromyalgia is a condition in which the person feels they hurt all over, including painful muscles and joints. And it can give other symptoms such as tiredness, headaches and depression. As with IBS, it is a diagnosis of exclusion because there is no test for fibromyalgia and, like IBS, fibromyalgia is a problem of function rather than structure, as there is nothing wrong with any organs when you have it. It is estimated that people with IBS have a 40 per cent higher chance of having fibromyalgia compared to people without.[5] It is thought that the connection might be the hypersensitivity to pain, and that with IBS the sensitivity is happening in the muscles in the bowels but with fibromyalgia it is happening in muscles elsewhere in the body. Some people will experience both together.

There are prescription drugs available for fibromyalgia that centre on controlling neurotransmitters like serotonin which are similar to some of the antidepressants being given for IBS (see page 238). There is also research on dietary interventions using similar strategies as for IBS as detailed in this book, with an interesting study on patients with fibromyalgia who also had IBS.[6] They were asked to remove both MSG (monosodium glutamate) and aspartame (an artificial sweetener) from their diet for four weeks. At the end of the four weeks an overwhelming 84 per cent of the patients said that over 30 per cent of their symptoms had resolved.[7] I suggest you try this yourself and see if it makes a difference.

CHRONIC FATIGUE SYNDROME (CFS)

Many chronic fatigue sufferers experience IBS symptoms as well as the exhaustion and muscle pain that characterize the syndrome. And again, as with IBS, it ends up as a diagnosis of exclusion because there is no definite test for CFS. Both IBS and CFS can be triggered by another illness, such as the flu, and as with fibromyalgia there are suggestions that an imbalance of serotonin may play a part, in the gut for IBS and in the brain for both CFS and fibromyalgia. It is also thought that stress plays a huge part in fibromyalgia, chronic fatigue and also IBS, so pay particular attention to the section on stress in Chapter 7 (see page 152).

Interesting research has looked at food hypersensitivity in relation to IBS, fibromyalgia and chronic fatigue. A group of patients who felt they had food hypersensitivity were assessed for IBS, fibromyalgia and chronic fatigue. All but one of the patients had IBS, 85 per cent of them had fibromyalgia and 71 per cent, chronic fatigue. No IgE allergies (page 44) were picked up in any of the patients but over 25 per cent had fat malabsorption.[8] The researchers state 'The comorbid triad of IBS, chronic fatigue, and musculoskeletal pain is striking and may point to a common underlying cause.'

So I strongly urge you to follow the recommendations in this book as what before might have seemed like unconnected conditions may all have the same underlying cause. You have nothing to lose by putting my nutritional recommendations into place and everything to gain.

CONCLUSION

AN END TO IBS

I hope that by reading this book you have both the realistic hope that you can discover the cause of your IBS and also a practical plan so that you can alleviate your symptoms and begin to build up the strength of your gut once again. For some people it might be a case of accepting that a particular food group like dairy or gluten must be avoided and then exploring all the really good alternatives that are now available. Or you may have realized that a bout of food poisoning triggered your IBS, have been tested and are now using supplements to rebalance the bacteria in your gut.

I do know that many people find it hard to stay with their healthy new IBS-free way of living indefinitely; sometimes life can put some pretty big obstacles in the way. So I've put together a few reminders that I hope will spur you on to keep putting your health first, because when we are feeling well we can cope so much better with all aspects of life, and we can really enjoy food rather than falling back into that negative pattern.

KEEP AN EYE OUT

Giving your body time to heal will allow your energy levels to return and I hope, in turn, your general sense of wellbeing and optimism will rise too. Really appreciate these feelings, try not to take them for granted, as they will help you see your new IBS-free lifestyle in a really positive light, rather than as something that is hard or that has taken something away.

When it comes to IBS your body will tell you straight away if things are not quite right. Be aware of how you feel each day, and whether foods in your diet are starting to creep up to levels that are putting your digestion under a little too much strain again.

If you are experiencing a stressful period in your life then take care to eat very simply and opt for foods that you know are comforting to your digestion rather than challenging. Often when stressed we might associate comfort food with sugar or fat, but they end up making us feel worse. If you feel stressed, pick up the book again and read through Chapter 7 to remind yourself of all the ways you can relax without reaching for those drinks and foods that drain your energy and can start up the pattern of IBS once again.

Remember to take time for meals rather than rush them. Don't eat while sitting at the computer, and always have healthy snacks on hand so that you don't get too hungry and end up grabbing whatever food is available, even when you know it's not good for your IBS.

It can be very difficult when you go out with friends or family to not be tempted by lots of foods that might trigger your symptoms, such as a slice of cake, a cream tea or pizza. I would say that it's a good idea to find a few weeks during which you can really allow your gut to have a break and heal without these sorts of challenges. And then you can see if just a little is OK for you or whether it's not worth it. Nowadays there are usually some delicious alternatives on most menus that mean you can still have a great time without suffering afterwards.

If you find that you are still panicking or worrying that you might become ill, even if your gut is feeling much better, then do consider whether a few sessions of CBT therapy might be just what you need to break this pattern of generalization. It's amazing what a big part our minds play when it comes to our bodies and with IBS people can bring on symptoms by worrying so much about them.

Don't fall into eating a very narrow diet. It is so important with IBS to not eat too much of anything as you might develop a sensitivity. For example if you are no longer eating dairy foods then don't just have soya milk as an alternative but also try oat, rice and nut milks too.

Always try to eat natural and, where possible, organic foods. When we know what's in our food then we can stay in relaxed control.

Remember that supplements can be very helpful. I recommend a good multivitamin and mineral, vitamin C and Omega 3 fish oils for everyone. Plus you might want to top up your good bacteria every now and then with a course of probiotics or soothe a minor irritation with aloe vera. Get to know which supplements work the best for you so that when you have the first signs of digestive disturbance you can take a natural supplement, as well as simplifying your diet for a few days.

Likewise if you find you have just a specific symptom starting to reappear then have another look at Chapter 8 and all the common digestive disorders. For example if you are feeling bloated you might simply need to release some water retention. Or you might need some quick tips on how to soothe heartburn after eating something you didn't realize would affect you.

MY TOP 10 IBS TIPS TO REMEMBER

1. Avoid caffeine and reduce your intake of alcohol.
2. Drink plenty of other fluids like water and herbal tea, little and often throughout the day – it makes such a difference to your digestion to keep well hydrated.
3. Keep your blood sugar balanced by eating regular and not too big meals, chew well and eat slowly in a relaxed frame of mind.
4. Avoiding wheat is a good idea for nearly all IBS sufferers. If you do have bread, then freshly baked on the premises with no additives or preservatives is best, as are more unusual grains like spelt.
5. Reduce your intake of saturated fats from meat and dairy.
6. Avoid sugar where possible.
7. Read food labels and avoid sorbitol, artificial sweeteners and added sugar or fructose.
8. Exercise.
9. Develop your own relaxation techniques.
10. Of all the 'extra' supplements I recommend taking a pro-biotic supplement more often than any other.

A FINAL WORD

A report published in 2011 asked the question 'IBS: what do patients really want?' and it concluded that what patients with IBS want is 'not only a competent but also a caring healthcare provider. They value relationship qualities of care as highly as they value knowledge and technical skills. It is becoming more apparent that not eliciting or redressing what patients want carries a high cost to human experience in health care spending. If the saying "people don't care how much you know until they know how much you care" is true, then healthcare professionals have an obligation to respond to patients' expectations for care, because care is what our patients both want and need.'[1]

So follow the recommendations in this book because they have come out of thirty years of experience of working with and caring for patients. I very much hope that you can see that you don't have to put up with your IBS symptoms, even though you might have been told before that you 'just have to live with them'. And if you feel that you need more individual help to guide you through the tests and how to implement the food aspects then do come into one of my clinics (see Useful Resources, page 207).

I do appreciate that it is not easy to make dramatic changes to the way you eat or live but you will be surprised at the improvement in your IBS and general digestive symptoms that can happen in a short space of time. You have got nothing to lose (apart from all your IBS symptoms!) and everything to gain. I know from years of working with patients in the clinic that my methods do work. You can get your life back, be free from discomfort and be able to travel and go wherever you want to without being anxious or on red alert the whole time. That sense of freedom is so worthwhile.

Your life, and your health, is very much in your hands.

Wishing you the best of health,

Marilyn

USEFUL RESOURCES

THE DR MARILYN GLENVILLE PHD CLINICS
NATURAL HEALTHCARE FOR WOMEN

Consultations

If you would like to have a consultation (either in person or by telephone), then please feel free to phone my clinic for an appointment.

All of the qualified nutritionists who work in my three UK clinics (and three in Ireland) have been trained by me in my specific approach to women's healthcare including, of course, IBS.

The clinics are located at the following addresses.

UK

- Viveka, St John's Wood, London
- The Medical Chambers, Kensington, London
- The Dr Marilyn Glenville Clinic, Tunbridge Wells, Kent

To book a personal or telephone appointment at any of these clinics, or for more information, please contact us at:

The Dr Marilyn Glenville Clinic
14 St John's Road
Tunbridge Wells
Kent TN4 9NP

Tel: 0870 5329244 / Fax: 0870 5329255
Int. Tel: ++44 1 892 515905 / Fax: ++ 44 1 892 515914
Email: health@marilynglenville.com
Website: www.marilynglenville.com

Ireland
- Dublin, Galway and Cork

To book a personal or telephone appointment at any of these clinics, or for more information, please contact us at:

Tel: 01 402 0777
www.marilynglenville.ie

WORKSHOPS AND TALKS

For a list of workshops and talks I will be presenting, please see my website www.marilynglenville.com. If you would like to organize a workshop or talk near you for me to come along, then call my clinic and ask for information about how to do this.

SUPPLEMENTS AND TESTS

The Natural Health Practice (NHP) is my supplier of choice for all the supplements and tests mentioned in this book. They only carry products that I use in my clinics and are in the correct form, the right dosage levels and use the highest-quality ingredients. For more information, please contact:

The Natural Health Practice
Website: www.naturalhealthpractice.com
Tel: 0845 8800915
Int. Tel: ++ 44 1 892 507598

FREE HEALTH TIPS

If you would like to receive my exclusive Health Tips by email, drop me a line at health@marilynglenville.com. Just mention 'Free Health Tips' in the subject line and you will be added to my special list to receive regular health tips and other useful information.

NOTES

Introduction
1. Hayee, B. and Forgacs, I., 'Psychological approach to managing irritable bowel syndrome', *BMJ*, **334** (2007), 7603, 1105–9

Chapter 1: What is IBS?
1. Spiller, R. *et al.*, 'Guidelines on IBS mechanisms and practical management', *Gut*, **56** (2007), 12, 1770–98
2. Drossman, D.A. *et al.*, 'A prospective assessment of bowel habit in irritable bowel syndrome in women: defining an alternator', *Gastroenterology*, **128** (2005), 3, 580–9
3. Ruigomez, A. *et al.*, 'Risk of IBS after an episode of bacterial gastroenteritis in general practice: influence of comorbidities', *Clin Gastroenterol Hepatol*, **5** (2007), 4, 465–9
4. Maxwell, P.R. *et al.*, 'Antibiotics increase functional abdominal symptoms', *Am J Gastroenterol*, **97** (2002), 1, 104–8
5. Hviid, A. I., 'Antibiotic use and inflammatory bowel diseases in childhood', *Gut*, **60** (2011), 1, 49–54
6. Payne, S., 'Sex, gender and irritable bowel syndrome: Making the connections', *Gender Medicine*, **1** (2004), 1, 18–28
7. Cain, K.C. *et al.*, 'Abdominal pain impacts quality of life in women with irritable bowel syndrome', *Am J Gastroenterol*, **101** (2006), 1, 124–32
8. Houghton, L.A. *et al.*, 'The menstrual cycle affects rectal sensitivity in patients with IBS but not healthy volunteers', *Gut*, **50** (2002), 4, 471–4
9. Tsynman, D.N. *et al.*, 'Treatment of irritable bowel syndrome in women', *Gastroenterol Clin North Am*, **40** (2011), 2, 265–90

211

10. Ruigomez, A. *et al.*, 'Is HRT associated with an increased risk of IBS?', *Maturitas*, **44** (2003), 2, 133–40

11. Heitkemper, M.M. and Chang, L., 'Do fluctuations in ovarian hormones affect gastrointestinal symptoms in women with irritable bowel syndrome', *Gend Med*, **6** (2009), Suppl 2, 152–67

12. Altman, G. *et al.*, 'Increased symptoms in female IBS patients with dysmenorrhea and PMS', *Gastroenterol Nurs*, **29** (2006), 1, 4–11

13. Olafsdottir, L.B. *et al.*, 'Natural history of irritable syndrome in women and dysmenorrhea: a 10 year follow up study', *Gastroenterol Res Pract*, (2012), March 14, published online ahead of publication

14. Khashan, A.S. *et al.*, 'Increased risk of miscarriage and ectopic pregnancy among women with irritable bowel syndrome', *Clin Gastroenterol Hepatol*, (2012), ahead of publication

15. Chassany, O. *et al.*, 'Drug-induced diarrhoea', *Drug Saf*, **22** (2000), 1, 53–72

16. Lewis, S.J. and Heaton, K.W., 'Stool form scale as a useful guide to intestinal transit time', *Scand J Gastroenterol*, **32** (1997), 9, 920–4

Chapter 3: Your Medical Options

1. Hayee, B. and Forgacs, I., 'Psychological approach to managing irritable bowel syndrome', *BMJ*, **334** (2007), 7603, 1105–9

2. Pitz, M. *et al.*, 'Defining the predictors of the placebo response in irritable bowel syndrome', *Clin Gastroenterol Hepatol*, **3** (2005), 237–47

3. Halpert, A. and Goldena, E., 'Irritable bowel syndrome patients' perspectives on their relationships with healthcare providers', *Scand J Gastroenterol*, **46** (2011), 7–8, 823–30

4. Enck, P. *et al.*, 'The placebo response in functional bowel disorders: perspectives and putative mechanisms', *Neurogastroenterol Motil*, **17** (2005), 325–310

5. Ruepert, L. *et al.*, 'Bulking agents, antispasmodic and antidepressant medication for the treatment of irritable bowel syndrome', *Cochrane Database Syst Rev*, **8** (2011), CD003460

6. Ruepert, L. *et al.*, 'Bulking agents, antispasmodic and antidepressant medication for the treatment of irritable bowel syndrome', *Cochrane Database Syst Rev*, **8** (2011), CD003460

7. Snook, J. and Shepherd, H.A., 'Bran supplementation in the treatment of irritable bowel syndrome', *Aliment Pharmacol Ther*, **8** (1994), 511–14

8. Ruepert. L., 'Bulking agents, antispasmodic and antidepressant medication for the treatment of irritable bowel syndrome', *Cochrane Database Syst Rev*, **8** (2011), CD003460

9. Hayee, B. and Forgacs, I., 'Psychological approach to managing irritable bowel syndrome', *BMJ*, **334** (2007), 7603, 1105–9

10. Tack, J. *et al.*, 'A controlled crossover study of the selective serotonin reuptake inhibitor citalopram in irritable bowel syndrome', *Neurogastroenterology*, **55** (2006), 1095–1103

11. Evans, B.W. *et al.*, 'Tegaserod for the treatment of irritable bowel syndrome and chronic constipation', *Cochrane Database Sys Rev*, **4** (2007), CD 003960

12. Jones, R., 'Treatment of irritable bowel syndrome in primary care', *BMJ*, **337** (2008), a2213

Chapter 4: Nutritional Tests

1. Liberman, J.A. and Sicherer, S.H., 'Diagnosis of food allergy: epicutaneous skin tests, in vitro tests, and oral food challenge', *Curr Allergy Asthma Rep*, **11** (2011), 1, 58–64

2. Gerez, I.F. *et al.*, 'Diagnostic tests for food allergy', *Singapore Med*, **51** (2010), 1, 4–9

3. Mullin, G.E.T. *et al.*, 'Testing for food reactions: the good, the bad, and the ugly', *Nutr Clin Pract*, **25** (2010), 2, 192–9

4. Wilders-Truschnig, M. *et al.*, 'IgG antibodies against food antigens are correlated with inflammation and intima media thickness in obese juveniles', *Exp Clin Endocrinol Diabetes*, **116** (2008), 4, 241–5

5. Buhner, S. *et al.*, 'Activation of human enteric neurons by supernatants of colonic biopsy specimens from patients with IBS', *Gastroenterology*, **137** (2009), 4, 1425–34

6. Zhou, Q. *et al.*, 'Increased membrane permeability and hypersensitivity in the irritable bowel syndrome', *Pain*, **146** (2009), 1–2, 41–6

7. Hammerie, C.W. and Crowe, S.E., 'When to reconsider the diagnosis of irritable bowel syndrome', *Gastroenterol Clin North Am*, **40** (2011), 2, 291–307

8. Ruigomez, A. *et al.*, 'Risk of IBS after an episode of bacterial gastroenteritis in general practice: influence of comorbidities', *Clin Gastroenterol Hepatol*, **5** (2007), 4, 465–9

9. El-Salhy, M. *et al.*, 'The prevalence of coeliac disease in patients with IBS', *Mol Med Report*, **4** (2011), 3, 403–5

10. Volta, U. and De Giorgio, R., 'New understanding of gluten sensitivity', *Nat Rev Gasstroenterol Hepatol*, **9** (2012), 5, 295–9

11. Hogg-Kollars, S. *et al.*, 'Gluten sensitivity a new condition in the spectrum of gluten-related disorders', *Complete Nutrition*, **11** (2011), 4, July/August

12. Parker, T.J. *et al.*, 'Irritable bowel syndrome: is the search for lactose intolerance justified?', *Eur J Gastroenterol Hepatol*,**13** (2001), 3, 219–25

13. Pimentel, M. *et al.*, 'Breath testing to evaluate lactose intolerance in irritable bowel syndrome correlates with lactulose testing and may not reflect true lactose malabsorption', *Am J Gastroenterol*, **98** (2003), 12, 2700–4

14. Hammerie, C.W. and Crowe, S.E., 'When to reconsider the diagnosis of IBS', *Gastroenterol Clin North Am*, **40** (2011), 2, 291–307

15. Kyaw, M.H. and Mayberry, J.F., 'Fructose malabsorption: true condition or a variance from normality', *J Clin Gastroenterol*, **45** (2011), 16–21

Chapter 5: Eating to Beat IBS

1. Lacy, B.E. *et al.*, 'Irritable bowel syndrome: patients attitudes, concerns and level of knowledge', *Aliment Pharmacol Ther*, **25**(2007), 1329–41

2. Eswaran, S. *et al.*, 'Food: the forgotten factor in the irritable bowel syndrome', *Gastroenterol Clin North Am*, **40** (2011), 1, 141–620

3. Cordain, L. *et al.*, 'Origins and evolution of the Western diet: health implications for the 21st century', *Am J Clin Nutr*, **81** (2005), 341–54

4. Bijkerk, C.J. *et al.*, 'Systematic review: the role of different types of fibre in the treatment of irritable bowel syndrome', *Aliment Pharmacol Ther*, **19** (2004), 3, 245–51

5. Gwee, K.A., 'Irritable bowel syndrome in developing countries – a disorder of civilization or colonization', *Neurogastroenterol Motil*, **17** (2005), 1–8

6. Parker, T.J. *et al.*, 'Irritable bowel syndrome: is the search for lactose intolerance justified?', *Eur J Gastroenterol Hepatol*, **13** (2001), 3, 219–25

7. Devkota, S. *et al.*, 'Dietary-fat-induced taurocholic acid promotes pathobiont expansion and colitis in l10$^{-/-}$ mice', *Nature*, **487** (2012), 104–108

8. World Health Organization, Joint WHO/FAO Expert Consultation

'Diet, Nutrition and the Prevention of Chronic Diseases', 2003, WHO Technical Report Series 916

9. Vonk, R.J. *et al.*, 'Digestion of so-called resistant starch sources in the human small intestines', *Am J Clin Nutr*, **72** (2000), 432–38

10. Johnson, K.L. *et al.*, 'Resistant starch improves insulin sensitivity in metabolic syndrome', *Diabetic Medicine*, **27** (2010), 391–97

11. Grabitske, H.A. and Slavin, J.L., 'Gastrointestinal effects of low-digestible carbohydrates', *Crit Rev Food Sci Nutr*, **49** (2009), 4, 327–60

12. Marteau, P. and Flourie. B., 'Tolerance to low-digestible carbohydrates: symptomatology and methods', *Br J Nutri*, **85** (2001), Suppl 1, S17–21

13. Simopoulos, A.P., 'Evolutionary aspects of diet: the Omega 6/Omega 3 ratio and the brain', *Mol Neurobiol*, **44** (2011), 2, 203–15

14. Noddin, L. *et al.*, 'Irritable Bowel Syndrome and Functional Dyspepsia: Different Diseases or a Single Disorder With Different Manifestations?', *Med Gen Med*, **7** (2005), 3, 17

15. Welsh, J.A. *et al.*, 'Caloric sweetener consumption and dyslipidemia among US adults', *JAMA*, **303** (2010), 15, 1490–7

16. Gray, J. and Griffin, B., 'Eggs and dietary cholesterol – dispelling the myth', *Nutrition Bulletin*, **34** (2009), 66–70

17. Cassady, B.A. *et al.*, 'Mastication of almonds: effects of lipid bioaccessibility, appetite, and hormone response', *J Am Clin Nutr*, **89** (2009), 3, 794–800

18. Staudacher, H.M. *et al.*, 'Comparison of symptom response following advice for a diet low in fermentable carbohydrates (FODMAPs) versus standard dietary advice in patients with IBS', *J Hum Nutr Diet*, **24** (2011), 5, 487–95

19. Gibson, P.R. and Shepherd, S.J., 'Evidence-based dietary management of functional gastrointestinal symptoms: the FODMAP approach', *J Gastroenterol Hepatol*, **25** (2010), 2, 252–8

20. Blundell, J.E. and Hill, A.J., 'Paradoxical effects of an intense sweetener (aspartame) on appetite' *Lancet*, **1** (1986), 8489, 1092–3

21. Maher, T.J. and Wurtman, R.J., 'Possible neurologic effects of aspartame, a widely used food additive', *Environ Health Perspect*, **75** (1987), 53–7

22. Rao, S.S. *et al.*, 'Is coffee a colonic stimulant?', *Eur J Gastroenterol Hepatol*, **10** (1998), 2, 113–8

23. Burden, S., 'Dietary treatment of irritable bowel syndrome: current evidence and guidelines for future practice', *J Hum Nutr Diet*, **14** (2001), 3, 231–41

24. Crisp, T.M. *et al.*, 'Environmental endocrine disruption: An effects assessment and analysis', *Environ Health Perspect*, **106** (1998), Supp 1, 11–56

25. Holton, K.F. *et al.*, 'The effect of dietary glutamate on fibromyalgia and irritable bowel symptoms', *Clin Exp Rheumatol*, (2012), July 4, ahead of publication

26. Giovannucci, E., 'The Role of Insulin Resistance and Hyperinsulinemia in Cancer Causation', *Curr Med Chem*, **5** (2005), 1, 53–60

27. Kabat, G.C., 'Repeated measures of serum glucose and insulin in relation to postmenopausal breast cancer', *Int J Cancer*, **125** (2009), 11, 2704–10

Chapter 6: How to Use Supplements, Herbs and Natural Remedies

1. The Independent Food Commission's Food Magazine, (2005)

2. Shen, Y.H. and Nahas, R., 'Complementary and alternative medicine for treatment of irritable bowel syndrome', *Can Fam Physician*, **55** (Feb 2009), 2, 143–80

3. Ligaarden, S.C. and Farup, P.G., 'Low intake of vitamin B(6) is associated with irritable bowel syndrome symptoms', *Nutr Res*, **31** (2011), 5, 35661

4. Murakami, K. *et al.*, 'Association between dietary fibre, water and magnesium intake and functional constipation among young Japanese women', *Eur J Clin Nutr*, **61** (2007), 616–22

5. Pearce, S.H. and Cheetham, T.D., 'Diagnosis and management of vitamin D deficiency', *BMJ*, **340** (2010), 7738, 142–47

6. Nowson, C.A. and Margerison, C., 'Vitamin D intake and vitamin D status of Australians', *Med J Aust*, **177** (2002), 3, 149–52

7. Narula, N. and Marshall, J.K., 'Management of inflammatory bowel disease with vitamin D: beyond bone health', *J Crohns Colitis*, (2011), Nov 25, ahead of publication

8. Yashodhara, B.M. *et al.*, 'Omega 3 fatty acids: a comprehensive review of their role in health and disease', *Postgrad Med J*, **85** (2009), 1000, 84–90

9. Buhner, S. *et al.*, 'Activation of human enteric neurons by supernatants of colonic biopsy specimens from patients with IBS', *Gastroenterology*, **137** (2009), 4, 1425–34

10. Cappello, G. *et al.*, 'Peppermint oil (Mintoil) in the treatment of irritable bowel syndrome: a prospective double blind placebo-controlled randomised trial', *Dig Liver Dis*, **39** (2007), 6, 530–6

11. Barbara, G. *et al.*, 'Probiotics and irritable bowel syndrome: rationale and clinical evidence for their use', *J Clin Gastroenterol*, **42** (2008), Suppl 3 Pt 2, S214–7

12. Parkes, G.C. *et al.*, 'Treating irritable bowel syndrome with probiotics: the evidence', *Proc Nutr Soc*, **69** (2010), 2, 187–94

13. Calder, P.C. *et al.*, 'Inflammatory disease processes and interactions with nutrition', *B J Nutr*, **101** (2009), Supp 1–45

14. Botschinsky, B. *et al.*, 'A review of the evidence available for the use and effectiveness of probiotic drinks and supplements for the treatment of irritable bowel syndrome', *Int J Probiotics and Prebiotics*, **6** (2011), 1, 21–38

15. Ryecroft, C.E. *et al.*, 'A comparative in vitro evaluation of the fermentation properties of prebiotic oligosaccharides', *J Appl Microbiol*, **91** (2001), 878–87

16. Whelan, K., 'Probiotics and prebiotics in the management of irritable bowel syndrome: a review of recent clinical trials and systematic reviews', *Curr Opin Clini Nutr Metab Care*, **14** (2011), 6, 581–7

17. Kolida, S. and Gibson, G.R., 'Synbiotics in health and disease', *Annu Rev Food Sci Technol*, **2** (2011), 373–93

18. Islam, M.S. *et al.*, 'Anti-inflammatory effects of phytosteryl ferulates in colitis induced by dextran sulphate sodium in mice', *Br J Pharmacol*, **154** (2008), 4, 812–24

19. Czerucka, D. *et al.*, 'Review article: yeast as probiotics – Saccharomyces boulardii', *Aliment Pharmacol Ther*, **26** (2007), 6, 767–78

20. Dinleyici, E.C. *et al.*, 'Effectiveness and safety of Saccharomyces boulardii for actute infectious diarrhoea', *Expert Opin Biol Ther*, **12** (2012), 4, 395–410

21. Buts, J.P. *et al.*, 'Saccharomyces boulardii: basic science and clinical applications in gastroenterology', *Gastroenterol Clin North Am*, **34** (2005), 3, 515–32

22. Choi, C.H. *et al.*, 'A randomised, double blind, placebo controlled multicentre trial of saccharomyces boulardii in irritable bowel syndrome: effect on quality of life', *J Clin Gastroenterol*, **45** (2011), 8, 679–83

23. Nievergelt, A. *et al.*, 'Identification of serotonin 5-HT1A receptor partial agonists in ginger', *Bioorganic and Medicinal Chemistry*, **18** (2010), 9, 3345–51

24. Hawrelak, J.A. and Myers, S.P., 'Effects of two natural medicine formulations on irritable bowel syndrome symptoms: a pilot study', *J Altern Complement Med*, **16** (2012), 10, 1065–71

25. Hawrelak, J.A. and Myers, S.P., 'Effects of two natural medicine formulations on irritable bowel syndrome symptoms: a pilot study', *J Altern Complement Med*, **16** (2012), 10, 1065–71

26. Cappello, G. *et al.*, 'Peppermint oil (Mintoil) in the treatment of irritable bowel syndrome: a prospective double blind placebo-controlled randomised trial', *Dig Liver Dis*, **39** (2007), 6, 530–6

27. Bundy, R. *et al.*, 'Turmeric extract may improve irritable bowel syndrome symptomology in otherwise healthy adults: a pilot study', *J Altern Complement Med*, **10** (2004), 6, 1015–8

28. Bundy, R. *et al.*, 'Artichoke leaf extract reduces symptoms of irritable bowel syndrome and improves quality of life in otherwise healthy volunteers suffering from concomitant dyspepsia: a subset analysis', *J Altern Complement Med*, **10** (2004), 4, 667–9

29. Hutchings, H.A. *et al.*, 'A Randomised, Cross-Over, Placebo-Controlled Study of Aloe vera in Patients with Irritable Bowel Syndrome: Effects on Patient Quality of Life', *ISRN Gastroenterol*, (2011), Epub 2010, ahead of print publication Oct 11

30. Piper, W., 'Yeast superoxide dismutase mutants reveal a pro-oxidant action of weak organic acid food preservatives', *Free Radic Biol Med*, **27** (1999), 11–12, 1219–27

31. Grimbergen, G.W., 'A double blind test for determination of intolerance to fluoridated water, Preliminary report', *Fluoride*, 7 (1974), 3, 146–52

32. Petraborg, H.T., 'Hydrofluorosis in the fluoridated Milwaukee area', *Fluoride*, **10** (1977), 4, 165–68

33. Gupta, I.P. *et al.*, 'Fluoride as a possible aetiological factor in non-ulcer dyspepsia', *J Gastroenterol Hepatol*, **4** (1992), 355–9

34. Das, T.K. *et al.*, 'Toxic effects of chronic fluoride ingestion on the upper gastrointestinal tract', *J Clin Gastroenterol*, **18** (1994), 3, 194–9 and Susheela, A.K., Das, T.K. and Gupta, I.P., 'Fluoride ingestion and its correlation with gastrointestinal discomfort', *Fluoride*, **25** (1992), 5–22

35. National Research Council, 'Fluoride in drinking water: A Scientific Review of EPA's Standards', National Academies Press, 2006, Washington DC

36. Medical Research Council working group report: Water fluoridation and health, 2002
37. National Research Council, 'Fluoride in drinking water: A Scientific Review of EPA's Standards', National Academies Press, 2006, Washington DC
38. Chanine, L. *et al.*, 'The effect of sodium lauryl sulphate on recurrent aphthous ulcers: a clinical study', *Compend Contin Educ Dent*, **18** (1997), 12, 1238–40
39. Linde, K. *et al.*, 'St John's wort for major depression', *Cochrane Database Syst Rev*, **4** (2008), CD000448
40. Heaney, R.P. *et al.*, 'Vitamin D(3) is more potent than vitamin D(s) in humans', *J Clin Endocrinol Metab*, **96** (2011), 3, E447–52
41. Dwyer, A.V. *et al.*, 'Herbal medicines, other than St. John's Wort, in the treatment of depression: a systematic review', *Altern Med Rev*, **16** (2011), 1, 40–9
42. Olsson, E.M. *et al.*, 'A randomised double-blind, placebo-controlled, parallel-group study of the standardised extract shr-5 of the roots of Rhodiola rosea in the treatment of subjects with stress-related fatigue', *Planta Med*, **75** (2009), 2, 105–12
43. Edwards, D. *et al.*, 'Therapeutic Effects and Safety of Rhodiola rosea Extract WS® 1375 in Subjects with Life-stress Symptoms – Results of an Open-label Study', *Phytother Res*, (2012), Jan 6
44. Manheimer, E. *et al.*, 'Acupuncture for treatment of irritable bowel syndrome', *Cochrane Database Syst Rev*, **5** (2012), CD005111

Chapter 7: Stress, Emotions and Exercise

1. Konturek, P.C. *et al.*, 'Stress and the gut: pathophysiology, clinical consequences, diagnostic approach and treatment options', *J Physiol Pharmacol*, **62** (2011), 6, 591–9
2. Lee, O.Y., 'Psychosocial factors and visceral hypersensitivity in IBS', *Korean J Gastroenterol*, **47** (2006), 2, 111–9
3. van der Veek, P.P. *et al.*, 'Clinical trial: short- and long-term benefit of relaxation training for irritable bowel', *Aliment Pharmacol Ther*, **26** (2007), 6, 943–52
4. Lackner, J.M. *et al.*, 'Psychological treatments for IBS: a systematic review and meta-analysis', *J Consult Clin Psychol*, **72** (2004), 1100–13

5. Gaylord, S.A. *et al.*, 'Mindfulness Training Reduces the Severity of Irritable Bowel Syndrome in Women: Results of a Randomized Controlled Trial', *Am J Gastroenterol*, **106** (2011), 9, 1678–88

6. Lindfors, P. *et al.*, 'Long-term effects of hypnotherapy in patients with refractory irritable bowel syndrome', *Scand J Gastroenterol*, **47** (2012), 4, 414–20

7. Gonsalkorale, W.M. *et al.*, 'Long term benefits of hypnotherapy for IBS', *Gut*, **52** (2003), 1623–9

8. Keefer, L. and Blanchard, E.B., 'The effects of relaxation response meditation on the symptoms of irritable bowel syndrome: results of a controlled treatment study', *Behav Res Ther*, **39** (2001), 801–811

9. Keefer, L. and Blanchard, E.B., 'A one year follow-up of relaxation response meditation as a treatment for irritable bowel syndrome', *Behav Res Ther*, **40** (2002), 541–54

10. Panossian, A. and Wilkman, G., 'Evidence-based efficacy of adaptogens in fatigue and molecular mechanisms related to their stress-protective activity', *Curr Clin Pharmacol*, **4** (2009), 3, 198–219

11. Vuong, Q.V. *et al.*, 'L-theanine: properties, synthesis and isolation from tea', *J Sci Food Agric*, **91** (2011), 11, 1931–9

12. Patel, S.R. *et al.*, 'Association between reduced sleep and weight gain in women', *Am J Epidemiol*, **164** (2006), 10, 947–54

13. Vege, S.S. *et al.*, 'Functional gastrointestinal disorders among people with sleep disturbances: a population-based study', *Mayo Clin Proc*, **79** (2004), 12, 1501–6

14. Bellini, M. *et al.*, 'Evaluation of latent links between irritable bowel syndrome and sleep quality', *World J Gastroenterol*, **17** (2011), 46, 5089–96

15. Chen, C.L. *et al.*, 'Evidence for altered anorectal function in irritable bowel syndrome patients with sleep disturbance', *Zhonghua Nei Ke Za Zhi*, **49** (2011), 7, 587–90

16. Jarrett, M. *et al.*, 'Sleep disturbance influences gastrointestinal symptoms in women with irritable bowel syndrome', *Dig Dis Sci*, **45** (2000), 5, 952–9

17. Johannesson, E. *et al.*, 'Physical activity improves symptoms in irritable bowel syndrome: a randomized controlled trial', *Am J Gastroenterol*, **106** (2011), 915–922

18. Fujiwara, Y. *et al.*, 'Cigarette smoking and its association with overlapping gastroesophageal reflux disease, functional dyspepsia or irritable bowel syndrome', *Intern Med*, **50** (2011), 21, 2443–7

Chapter 8: Common Digestive Problems

1. Carter, D. and Beer-Gabel, M., 'Lower urinary tract symptoms in chronically constipated women', *Int Urogynecol*, (2012), May 16, ahead of print publication
2. Marshall, J.K. *et al.*, 'Intestinal permeability in patients with irritable bowel syndrome after a waterborne outbreak of acute gastroenteritis in Walkerton, Ontario', *Aliment Pharmacol Ther*, **20** (2004), 1317–22
3. Thabane, M. *et al.*, 'Systematic review and meta-analysis: The incidence and prognosis of post-infectious irritable bowel syndrome', *Aliment Pharmacol Ther*, **26** (2007), 535–44
4. Thabane, M. and Marshall, J.K., 'Post-infectious irritable bowel syndrome', *World J Gastroenterol*, **15** (2009), 29, 3591–6
5. Cole, J.A. *et al.*, 'Migraine, fibromyalgia and depression among people with IBS: a prevalence study', *BMC Gastroenterol*, **6** (2006), 26
6. Arranx, L.I. *et al.*, 'Fibromyalgia and nutrition, what do we know?', *Rheumatol Int*, **30** (2010), 11, 1417–27
7. Holton, K.F. *et al.*, 'The effect of dietary glutamate on fibromyalgia and irritable bowel symptoms', *Clin Exp Rheumatol*, (2012), July 4, ahead of publication
8. Berstad, A. *et al.*, 'Functional bowel symptoms, fibromyalgia and fatigue: A food-induced triad?', *Scand J Gastroenterol*, (2012), May 18

Conclusion

1. Halpert, A., 'Irritable bowel syndrome: what do patients really want?', *Curr Gastroenterol Rep*, **13** (2011), 4, 331–5

INDEX